CANCER ETIOLOGY, DIAGNOSIS AND TREATMENTS

BLADDER CANCER

RISK FACTORS, EMERGING TREATMENT STRATEGIES AND CHALLENGES

CANCER ETIOLOGY, DIAGNOSIS AND TREATMENTS

Additional books in this series can be found on Nova's website under the Series tab.

Additional e-books in this series can be found on Nova's website under the e-book tab.

CANCER ETIOLOGY, DIAGNOSIS AND TREATMENTS

BLADDER CANCER

RISK FACTORS, EMERGING TREATMENT STRATEGIES AND CHALLENGES

SAMANTHA HAGGERTY
EDITOR

New York

For permission to use material from this book please contact us:
Telephone 631-231-7269; Fax 631-231-8175
Web Site: http://www.novapublishers.com

Library of Congress Cataloging-in-Publication Data

ISBN: 978-1-63321-666-2

Library of Congress Control Number: 2014946012

Published by Nova Science Publishers, Inc. † New York

CONTENTS

PREFACE

Bladder cancer is the fifth most common form of cancer worldwide and is mainly prevalent in developed countries. It is thought to arise through two distinct pathways: the noninvasive and the invasive. The noninvasive pathway gives rise to a superficial papillary carcinoma that is characterized by activating mutations in oncogenes such as H-ras, FGFR3 and PI3K. This pathway is rarely lethal as superficial papillary carcinomas can be readily removed through transurethral resection. However, 15% of noninvasive urothelial tumors can transform into invasive carcinomas and have high recurrence (80% of the cases) that requires intensive surveillance and repetitive treatment. This book discusses the risk factors of bladder cancer, as well as the emerging treatment strategies and challenges.

Chapter 1 – Epithelial tumors contain a heterogeneous population of cells that can be characterized by differences in their histopathology as well as functional properties. Emerging evidence supports the existence of tumor-initiating cells (T-ICs) or cancer stem cells (CSCs), which can self-renew and differentiate into progeny cells and subsequently result in the observed cellular and functional heterogeneity of epithelial tumors. Bladder cancer is the second most common urological malignancy and its invasive subtype remains notorious for resistance to conventional therapeutics and poor prognosis. Recent studies have focused on the identification and characterization of bladder cancer stem cells (CSCs) that are implicated in cancer recurrence and chemotherapy resistance, in the hope of early diagnosis and improved treatment. In this review, the authors discuss the existence of CSCs in general, as well as specifically in bladder cancers with focuses on the development of normal urothelial stem cells, origins of bladder CSCs, regulatory signaling pathways involved and therapeutic approaches to target CSCs. They believe that a better understanding of bladder CSCs as well as the development of novel targeting strategies should greatly benefit bladder cancer patients suffering from both non-invasive and invasive subtypes. Both approaches should be of great clinical relevance because they can significantly contribute to the development of new diagnostic markers and therapeutic targets.

Chapter 2 – Bladder carcinoma (BC) is the second most common malignancy of the urinary tract in males after prostate cancer. Diagnosis is usually subsequent to patients' report of blood in the urine (macrohematuria) frequently without pain. Yet, macrohematuria may be also associated to other bladder conditions such as stones, infections, or benign tumors, and its presence may be intermittent or not assessable without a specific test (urinalysis), thus bleeding is sometimes diagnosed serendipitously during routine checkups. Bleeding in BC is caused by the presence of fragile tissue, but this is related neither to the stage nor to the extension of the neoplastic lesion. Other non-exclusive symptoms involve irritative bladder behaviors, such as changes in urination frequency, dysuria and urgency; in case of large cancers, lower back pain or inability to urinate may be present. Also in these situations, the abovementioned symptoms may be associated to other clinical conditions not related to BC. Thus, it is extremely important to verify its presence and to perform an accurate differential diagnosis. *Hearing* the patient, and accurately report all symptoms and possible risk factors during anamnesis (smoking, professional exposure to chemicals, persistent phlogosis) is thus crucial to address him/her to a specialist for more specific analyses. A reliable assessment of BC presence and stage may be obtained mainly by a *visual*, direct analysis of the bladder followed by subsequent evaluation of a specialist urologist, using cystoscopy, tomography, ultrasonography and urinary cytology. These techniques will be analyzed here and newest frontiers in their development will be explained. The authors will show an overview of the most used biological markers of BC traceable inside urine and used for both diagnosis and stadiation purposes, allowing to *taste* urine content and helping in both diagnosis and possible cure. They will illustrate the mechanism of action of a palpation device, that allows differentiating normal and cancer samples by *touching* a bioptic specimen. The authors will also describe a recently developed technique able to *smell* volatile molecules from the urine of patients and to help in diagnosis. Finally, they will describe recent advances in BC diagnostics obtained by electrical impedance spectroscopy.

Chapter 3 – Lower urinary tract malignancies are very rare in pediatric age and highly uncommon in the first two decades of life; indeed, according to most available reports, their incidence among all affected patients if far lower that 1%. In fact, the sum of all patients for all bladder tumours in available scientific literature is just a few hundreds. These pathologies resemble in some instances their adult counterparts, such as painless macroscopic haematuria as first symptom, the males are more affected than females, the familiarity, the relationship with specific chemicals such as those linked to pollution. Nonetheless, there are other aspects of bladder cancers (BC) in children that show specific characteristics: (i) pediatric BC are usually unifocal; (ii) despite delayed diagnosis due to the unexpected pathology, consequently driving towards a different initial diagnosis, children usually show lower grade and stage cancers at presentation, compared to adults; (iii) their prognosis is, in general, relatively good compared to that of elder people; (iv) the recurrence rate is very low; (v) the tumors usually show an indolent behavior; (vi) although males are more affected, the male-to-female ratio shows an age-dependent value, with males being more affected at younger ages. Taken together, these facts suggest that BC in young patients is different from that of elderly people. Moreover, also its treatment needs a different approach, since in children and adolescents it is very important to preserve fertility and sexual performances. In this report, similarities and differences in BC between young and adults will be discussed, and alternative therapeutic approaches will be illustrated.

Chapter 4 – Cancers can be considered as a group of diseases, where cells undergo an uncontrolled growth, and malignant tumors are formed. Between them, bladder cancer (BLC) is an aggressive type of cancer, which can propagate from the urinary bladder to other organs in the human body. BLC is the seventh most common cancer around the world, contributing with more than 4% of all deaths caused by cancers. A very good alternative in the battle against this serious disease is the use of chemotherapy. However, for the design of efficient anti-BLC agents, it is necessary to cover a huge space in terms of molecular diversity and complexity. Consequently, chemoinformatics could be a great ally, helping to rationalize the discovery of new and versatile anti-BLC drugs in terms of diminution of financial resources and time. Current computer-aided models are able to predict anti-BLC activity against only one biological target (protein, cancer cell line) by using very limited and homogenous datasets. On the other hand, there is no information related with the possible safety of anti-BLC agents which have been tested. In this chapter, the authors introduce a multi-tasking (mtk) chemoinformatic model for simultaneous prediction of anti-BLC activity and safety profiles such as ADMET (absorption, distribution, metabolism, elimination, toxicity) properties. At the same time, the authors provide two useful insights regarding the molecular patterns that can be responsible for the anti-BLC activity and/or ADMET properties. In this sense, they give a physicochemical and/or structural explanation about the molecular descriptors which entered in their mtk-chemoinformatic model, and how a defined biological effect can be enhanced. On the other hand, the authors show a procedure for the calculation and analysis of quantitative contributions of molecular fragments to the biological effects, which can be a useful guide for experts working in medicinal chemistry and pharmaceutical sciences.

Chapter 5 – Bladder cancer (BC) is a heterogeneous disease with 70% of patients presenting superficial tumours and 30% presenting muscle-invading disease with a high risk of death associated to metastasis. The diagnosis is carried out by urine cytology, whith high specificity but low sensitivity, and cystoscopy, an expensive and unpleasant procedure. Carcinoma *in situ* and other high grade non-muscle-invasive tumors are treated by intravesical administration of BCG or other chemotherapeutic agents, while the indication for muscle-invasive disease is radical cystectomy.

Human cells express a family of mitochondrial long non-coding RNAs (ncRNAs). One of these transcripts, the sense mitochondrial ncRNA or SncmtRNA, is expressed in normal proliferating cells and tumor cells but not in non-dividing cells. In addition, normal human proliferating cells express two antisense transcripts, ASncmtRNA-1 and ASncmtRNA-2. Strikingly however, the ASncmtRNAs are down-regulated in tumor cell lines as well as in tumor cells present in different types of human cancer, including BC. Therefore, the differential expression profile of these transcripts allows to detect cancer cells in biopsies and biological fluids.

Down-regulation of the ASncmtRNAs seems to be an important hallmark of cancer and, hypothetically, may also represent a general vulnerability of cancer cells. Indeed, knock-down of the ASncmtRNAs using antisense oligonucleotides (ASO) exerts negative effects on cell proliferation and viability of bladder cancer cell lines representing a novel therapeutic strategy for this disease. The authors discuss recent advances on the use of the mitochondrial ncRNAs as targets for diagnostic and therapeutic protocols of BC and its potential use in the clinic.

Chapter 6 – The majority (more than 90%) of malignant neoplasms arising in the bladder are pure urothelial (transitional cell) carcinomas, and the rest (less than 10%) consist of histological variants of bladder cancer, including urothelial carcinoma admixed with other histologic patterns (squamous/glandular differentiation, nested, microcystic, clear cell, plasmacytoid, lymphoepithelioma-like, micropapillary, sarcomatoid variants, etc.) and pure forms of non-urothelial carcinoma (squamous cell carcinoma, adenocarcinoma, small cell carcinoma, etc.). These histological variants of bladder cancer have been described in a number of case series for several years and have been recognized in the 2004 World Health Organization Classification of urothelial cancers. These histological variants of bladder cancer have clinical significance at various levels, including diagnostic, that is, recognition of the morphological variant is necessary in order to avoid diagnostic misinterpretations; prognostic for patient risk stratification; and therapeutic, where a diagnosis of a particular variant may be associated with the administration of a therapy distinctive from that used in conventional urothelial carcinoma. In this article, the authors will chiefly review the literature on the histological variants of urothelial carcinoma with a focus on the prognostic and therapeutic implications of histological variants for the management of patients with bladder cancer.

Chapter 7 – Cisplatin-based systemic chemotherapy is the gold standard approach for patients with advanced or metastatic urothelial carcinoma (UC). Combined chemotherapy with methotrexate, vinblastine, doxorubicin and cisplatin (MVAC), which was developed about 25 years ago, is an effective and frequently used modality for these life-threatening diseases. Recently, combined chemotherapy with gemcitabine and cisplatin (GC) has become another standard treatment for advanced UC. However, several limitations remain with MVAC and GC treatment. Long-term follow-up has revealed that overall survival or progression-free survival is poor, particularly with metastatic UC. There is no standard second-line treatment in patients with UC after the failure of cisplatin-based chemotherapy.

Multimodal treatment has become a standard of care for other kinds of malignancy. Combined chemotherapy with radiation for the treatment of advanced bladder cancer remains questionable, including whether this would eradicate local disease, eliminate potential micrometastases, and maintain the best quality of life possible without compromising survival.

In addition, new chemotherapy regimen, gemcitabine and paclitaxel, that is reacted with another antitumor mechanism will be effective for patients with advanced or metastatic UC who have previously been treated with MVAC. A gemcitabine and paclitaxel pharmacokinetic study showed that paclitaxel increased the accumulation of gemcitabine triphosphate, the active metabolite of gemcitabine

Furthermore, new approaches shall be taken, and one of them could be specific immunotherapy. A personalized peptide vaccination (PPV) protocol where at maximum four peptides were chosen from many candidate peptides based on pre-existing humoral immunity followed by vaccination. The authors reviewed here three novel approaches in patients with advanced or metastatic UC.

In: Bladder Cancer
Editor: Samantha Haggerty
ISBN: 978-1-63321-666-2

Chapter 1

CANCER STEM CELL (CSC) IN BLADDER MALIGNANCY

Jianmin Zhang*, Maxime Blijlevens and Nuo Yang
[1]Department of Cancer Genetics,
Roswell Park Cancer Institute, Elm &Carlton Streets, Buffalo, NY, US

ABSTRACT

Epithelial tumors contain a heterogeneous population of cells that can be characterized by differences in their histopathology as well as functional properties. Emerging evidence supports the existence of tumor-initiating cells (T-ICs) or cancer stem cells (CSCs), which can self-renew and differentiate into progeny cells and subsequently result in the observed cellular and functional heterogeneity of epithelial tumors. Bladder cancer is the second most common urological malignancy and its invasive subtype remains notorious for resistance to conventional therapeutics and poor prognosis. Recent studies have focused on the identification and characterization of bladder cancer stem cells (CSCs) that are implicated in cancer recurrence and chemotherapy resistance, in the hope of early diagnosis and improved treatment. In this review, we discuss the existence of CSCs in general, as well as specifically in bladder cancers with focuses on the development of normal urothelial stem cells, origins of bladder CSCs, regulatory signaling pathways involved and therapeutic approaches to target CSCs. We believe that a

* To whom correspondence should be addressed. Tel: 716-845-5929; Fax: 716-845-1698; E-mail: jianmin.zhang@roswellpark.org.

better understanding of bladder CSCs as well as the development of novel targeting strategies should greatly benefit bladder cancer patients suffering from both non-invasive and invasive subtypes. Both approaches should be of great clinical relevance because they can significantly contribute to the development of new diagnostic markers and therapeutic targets.

INTRODUCTION

Bladder cancer is the 5th most common form of cancer worldwide and is mainly prevalent in developed countries [1]. It is thought to arise through two distinct pathways: the noninvasive and the invasive. The noninvasive pathway gives rise to a superficial papillary carcinoma that is characterized by activating mutations in oncogenes such as H-ras, FGFR3 and PI3K [2]. This pathway is rarely lethal as superficial papillary carcinomas can be readily removed through transurethral resection. However, 15% of noninvasive urothelial tumors can transform into invasive carcinomas and have high recurrence (80% of the cases) that requires intensive surveillance and repetitive treatment.

The invasive pathway on the other hand generates carcinoma *in situ* (CIS), a flat, high-grade lesion characterized by loss-of-function mutation in tumor suppressor genes such as p53, RB and PTEN [1]. Invasive urothelial carcinoma is a more aggressive tumor type and often becomes metastatic with a poor prognosis and a 5-year survival rate of only 5%. Common chemotherapeutics in invasive bladder cancers involves cisplatin and mitomycin C, either with or without 5-fluorouracil. However, 90% of the patients eventually suffer from recurrence associated with cisplatin-resistance, manifesting a critical issue in the treatment of invasive bladder cancer. Moreover, resistance to mitomycin C and radiotherapy has been reported as well [3, 4].

Drug resistance, tumor recurrence and metastasis are common themes in bladder cancer as well as other malignancies. One explanation that has been explored extensively and intensively in the past couple of decades is the cancer stem cell (CSC) hypothesis [5]. The CSC model postulates a hierarchical organization of cells such that only a small subset is responsible for sustaining tumorigenesis and establishing the cellular heterogeneity inherent in the primary tumor [6]. This model has gained wide attention because it provides an explanation for resistance to both radiation and chemotherapy as well as tumor relapse. Here we review the existence of CSCs in general, as well as specifically in bladder cancers with focuses on the development of normal urothelial stem cells, origins of bladder CSCs, regulatory signaling pathways involved and therapeutic approaches to target CSCs.

THE EXSTENCE OF CSCS

CSCs were initially established in hematologic malignancies. The hematopoietic system is the best characterized somatic tissue with respect to stem-cell biology [7]. Cancer stem cells are readily detected in myelogenous leukemia (CML), acute myelogenous leukemia (AML) and acute lymphoblastic leukemia (ALL) [8-10]. Leukemic stem cells have displayed high turnover that could not be attributed to their inability to respond to cytostatic effects implemented by the immune system [11]. These so-called long-term culture-initiating cells (LTC-IC) were thought to have bypassed the inhibitory signals that regulate the cycle of normal stem cells [12]. Leukemia CSCs have well-described stem-cell phenotype and a quiescent cell cycle status, suggesting that conventional anti-proliferative cytotoxic treatment are unlikely to be effective for them [7].

In breast cancer, the CSC theory has been initially proposed to account for tumor heterogeneity and later expanded to describe that breast cancer heterogeneity results from the ability of different subsets of normal breast stem and progenitor cells to transform into distinct breast CSCs [13, 14]. Of note, in 2003, Al-Hajj et al., published a paper in which they demonstrated the existence of breast CSCs [15]. When they injected breast cancer cells into mice, only a small subset of these breast cancer cells had the ability to form a tumor. These tumor-initiating cells (TICs) or CSCs were further isolated as $CD44^{+}/CD24^{-}$, which has nowadays been widely accepted as reliable breast CSC markers.

In prostate cancer, a xenograft line of small-cell undifferentiated prostate carcinoma displayed common morphological features as well as the expression of carcinoembyronic antigen (CEA) to the donor tumor [16]. More recently, many other stem cell markers have been proposed for prostate cancer. For example, it was found that $CD166^{high}$ prostate CSCs were significantly more capable of forming tubules in xenografts, a measurement of tissue regeneration capacity [17]. Additionally, stem cells with a $Lin^{-}/Sca1^{+}/CD49^{high}$ (LSC^{high}) signature isolated from murine prostate gland were capable of initiating tumor growth in *Pten*-Null mice [18]. Furthermore, signaling pathways involved in normal development have also been shown to play a role in the self-renewal of prostate CSCs, such as the Wnt/Hedgehog/Notch pathway [19-21].

In brain tumors, CSCs exhibited the upregulation of genes implicated in normal neural stem cells and they could further differentiate into both neurons and ganglia, as often seen in brain tumors [22]. The so-called side-population (SP) cells have been isolated from a glioma cell line by Hoechst 33342 staining and shown to induce tumor formation in mice, thus confirmed as CSCs [23]. In addition, CD133 has been used to study CSCs in the nervous system and CD133+ cells were capable of producing tumors in the mouse brain [24]. However, further studies reported that $CD133^-$ cells could also give rise to glioblastomas [25, 26], pointing to a debatable role of CD133 as a sound brain CSC marker. Other CSC markers proposed for glioblastoma include SSEA-1, as it confers the self-renewal and multilineage potential as well as initiates tumor growth *in vivo*; and integrin α6 as its inhibition decreases the self-renewal and tumor formation potential of glioblastoma cells [27]. Similar to the prostate cancer, the Notch pathway has also been implicated in inducing the self-renewal of glioblastoma CSCs [28].

Normal Urothelial Stem Cells

The human bladder consists of several layers, i.e., adventitia, muscular layer, lamina propria and transitional epithelium (or urothelium) from outer to inner side. The urothelium is further composed of three distinct cellular layers: 1) a single layer of basal cells located just above the basement membrane, 2) multiple layers of intermediate cells and 3) the innermost layer of large, multinucleated umbrella cells sealed by tight junctions [29]. It has been hypothesized that a cellular hierarchy exists within the urothelium, in that urothelial stem cells reside in the basal cell layer and give rise to basal cells, intermediate cells as well as umbrella cells. Such hypothesis is supported by the observation that although the urothelium is slow-cycling, during tissue damage the bladder has an outstanding regenerative capacity, indicating the existence of urothelial stem cells. For example, it was shown that BrdU label-retaining cells, i.e., stem cells as they lost labelling relatively slow due to their quiescent nature, were localized in the basal cell layer. Furthermore, these cells could become highly proliferative and form colonies at great efficacy [30]. It was further identified that the proliferative capacity of urothelial cells decreased towards the bladder lumen [31]. In contrast, Castillo-Martin et al., postulated that basal cells and umbrella cells arise from different rather than common progenitor cells [1]. Their hypothesis is based on the observation that basal cells were p63 positive and displayed high-weight cytokeratins (CKs) 5, 10 and 14, whereas umbrella cells were p63 negative and displayed low-weight CK18 and CK20 as well as uroplakin (a molecule thought to regulate membrane permeability). p63 is a homolog of p53 and encodes for two main isoforms produced by alternative promoters, TAp63 and ΔNp63. ΔNp63 is involved in multiple functions during skin development and in adult stem/progenitor cell regulation [32]. In contrast, TAp63 has been mostly restricted to its apoptotic function and more recently as the guardian of oocyte integrity [33]. p63 is considered to be essential for the normal development of stratified epithelia including urothelium. Interestingly, Larsson et al., isolated clonogenic urothelial cells that were capable of differentiating into urothelium when implanted in the nude mice and p63 was found to correlate with their self-renewal capacity [34]. Taken together, it is also possible that urothelial stem cells are just $p63^+$ basal/intermediate-like cells capable of differentiating into $p63^-$ umbrella cells, as supported by the finding that ΔNp63-positive basal cells generated both intermediate and umbrella cells [35]. Nevertheless, with these two prevailing hypotheses to be yet confirmed, the identity of the bladder stem cells remains elusive.

Urothelial Cancer Stem Cells

The highly hierarchic human bladder anatomy and cytology implicates that similar hierarchy may exist within the bladder cancer development, mostly likely mediated by bladder CSCs. Indeed, bladder cancer exhibits dual-track carcinogenesis, i.e., it follows the direction of either invasive or non-invasive growth, leading to an interesting debate on whether these two carcinogenic pathways originate from a common yet later diverged CSC or from primarily distinct CSCs.

In accordance with the assumption that basal cells function as putative urothelial stem cells, several studies have proposed bladder CSCs to arise from this cell type. Dotsikas et al., showed antigenic similarity between basal cells of the normal urothelial and differentiated papillary urothelial carcinomas [36]. Normal basal urothelial cells, but not intermediate or umbrella cells, expressed CD44; and more interestingly, CD44 expression was highest in non-invasive papillary carcinomas and diminished in invasive carcinomas [37, 38]. In a tissue array examination of more than 300 bladder cancer specimens by immunohistochemistry, it was reported that the $CD44^+$ tumor cells often colocalized with CK5 and were mutually exclusive to CK20 expression, a pattern similar to that of normal bladder basal cells (lineage-CD44(+)CK5(+)CK20(-)). Of particular note, such cells constitute a tumor-initiating cell (TIC) population as defined functionally by their enriched ability to induce xenograft tumors *in vivo* [39].

As mentioned above, p63 is exclusively expressed in bladder basal but not umbrella cells; and high expression of p63 has also been reported in malignant but not normal bladder cell lines [40]. Indeed, data on the correlation between the p63 level and bladder malignancy have been controversial. Initial studies showed that loss of p63 in invasive bladder carcinomas was associated with poor prognosis and decreased survival [41, 42]. For example, Park et al., examined p63 expression in normal urothelium, low-grade papillary noninvasive (LPN) urothelial tumors and high-grade/invasive carcinomas using either an isoform-nonspecific or a ΔN-isoform-specific antibody. Intense nuclear p63 immunostaining was found in a majority of LPN tumors, whereas it was frequently impaired in high-grade or muscle-invasive carcinomas. At the mRNA level, ΔNp63 expression predominated over TAp63, and amounts of ΔNp63 mRNA correlated with the p63 immunoreactivity, confirming that ΔNp63 accounted for p63 expressed in urothelial tissues. In cultured cells, ΔNp63 was also expressed in low-grade tumor cells as well as normal urothelial cells, but undetectable in high-grade aggressive carcinoma cells. Thus, impaired ΔNp63 expression characterizes aggressive phenotypes of urothelial neoplasms [43]. In contrast, a more recent study demonstrated that decreased survival in muscle-invasive bladder carcinoma actually correlated with a high p63 expression [44]. Such discrepancy may be explained by the fact that basal cells express different isoforms of p63, i.e., TAp63 and ΔNp63. Nevertheless, further studies on the role of p63 as well as its isoforms in bladder tumorigenesis are in order.

In summary, both CD44+CK5+CK20- and CK17+CEACAM6- cells, which are generally believed to arise from basal cells, are capable of initiating tumors in xenograft and thus proposed as putative bladder cancer CSCs. Last, in an effort to solve the puzzle as to the origin of non-muscle invasive (NMI) and muscle-invasive (MI) bladder cancers, Dancik et al., developed a novel statistical framework to assess whether NMI and MI tumors arise from a distinct progenitor cell (DPC) or common progenitor cell. Their model favored the DPC hypothesis, which was further supported by an analysis of 874 patients. This study provides a paradigm shift in our understanding of bladder cancer biology that has significant diagnostic and therapeutic implications [37].

PATHTHWAYS REGULATING CSC FUNCTIONS

Elucidation of the signaling pathways that regulate the maintenance and survival of CSCs is important for the development of novel therapies. Many CSC subsets and normal tissue stem cells seem to share core regulatory genes and developmental pathways. In the hematopoietic system, there is evidence of constitutive activation of both the nuclear factor-kB (NF-kB) and phosphatidylinositol 3' (PI3) kinase signaling pathways in acute myeloid leukemia (AML) stem cells, whereas pharmacological inhibition of NF-kB or PI3 kinase reduced the growth of AML stem cells [45, 46]. The Wnt pathway also has been shown to play an important role in the self-renewal of leukemic stem cells (LSCs) in AML [47]. In chronic myeloid leukemia (CML), Hedgehog (Hh) signaling was identified to be essential for the maintenance and function of LSCs, as shown by two independent studies that loss of Smoothened (Smo), an essential component of the Hh pathway, impaired haematopoietic stem cell renewal and decreased induction of chronic CML by the BCR-ABL1 oncoprotein [48, 49]. Stem cell-driven epithelial homeostasis in the intestine is regulated by four key signaling pathways: Wnt, Notch and epidermal growth factor (EGF) maintain the epithelial stem cell status, whereas bone morphogenetic protein (BMP) activates cell differentiation [50]. Wnt signaling has emerged as one of the most affected pathways in intestinal malignancies, as many of these tumors acquire Wnt mutations that disrupt epithelial differentiation and stem cell homeostasis. For example, aberrant activation of Wnt genes, such as CTNNB1, or inactivation of the tumor suppressor Apc (adenomatous polyposis coli) (51, 52) often results in intestinal hyperplasia including adenomatous polyps and benign adenomas [53]. This occurs due to the nuclear accumulation of β-catenin and the consequent abnormal expansion of a transformed epithelia stem cell compartment [54].

The Hippo pathway coordinates cell proliferation, apoptosis and differentiation, and has emerged as a major regulator of organ development and regeneration [55]. The central components of the mammalian Hippo pathway are two transcription co-activators, YAP (yes associated protein) and TAZ (transcriptional co-activator with PDZ-binding motif; also known as WWTR1). Both are controlled by a kinase cascade that is sensitive to mechanosensory and cell polarity cues [56]. An important role of the Hippo pathway in embryonic stem cells (ESCs) was indicated from studies on TAZ in human ESCs in that TAZ knockdown impaired the maintenance of the pluripotent state [57]. Furthermore, murine ESC pluripotency was demonstrated to require YAP [58-60]. On the other hand, genetic study in mice indicated that YAP is important for governing the intestine stem cell (ISC) properties [61]. Overexpression of a nucleus-localized YAP mutant in the small intestine resulted in enhanced proliferation and consequent expansion of the ISC population, potentially through the crosstalk with the Wnt and Notch pathways [61].

Further mouse studies indicated that the Hippo pathway influences the epidermal stem cell fate and liver regeneration [62-64]. Of note, the acquisition of CSC-like properties has been linked to the epithelial-to-mesenchymal transition (EMT) in mammary tissues, and the combination of self-renewing abilities with migratory and invasive properties is suggested to drive aggressive cancers [65, 66]. Interestingly, it has been shown that both YAP and TAZ induced EMT and cellular transformation in breast epithelial cells [67, 68]. Moreover, TAZ has been found to be frequently overexpressed in high-grade breast cancers and confer breast CSC traits [69].

Therapeutic Strategies to Target CSCs

It has been widely believed that notorious cancer resistance to conventional therapies may result from the existence of CSCs [70, 71]. First, quiescent CSCs are missed by the strategies that only target highly proliferative tumor cells. Second, a common feature of CSCs is the expression of proteins associated with the efflux of xenobiotic toxins (e.g. multidrug resistant proteins and related members of the ATP-binding transporters). A wide range of cancer cells, particularly during relapse, express these proteins and thus providing resistance to many chemotherapeutic drugs [72].

One obvious approach to target cancer stem cells is through targeting their self-renewal pathways; however, cautions should be taken as to selectively ablate only CSCs without affecting normal stem cell functions. One example is targeting of the Hh pathway. Pharmacologic inhibition of the Hh pathway in human and mouse leukemias inhibited the expansion of imatinib-resistant CML [48, 49], although it will also be of crucial importance to determine the effects of these therapeutic agents on normal HSC function.

Meanwhile, active Hh signaling pathway has also been identified in glioblastoma CSCs, and inhibition with the Hh pathway inhibitor cyclopamine or siRNAs directed against the Hh pathway components resulted in the loss of tumorigenic potential [73-75]. Last, in breast cancer, the Hh pathway components are highly expressed in mammary stem/progenitor cells, and cyclopamine has been shown to specifically inhibit mammary stem self-renewal *in vitro* [76]. These encouraging results have led to further studies on the targeting of CSCs by Hh pathway inhibitors in various cancers, with some being tested in clinical trials [73].

Another promising approach to target CSCs is antibody-based therapy [7]. For example, it has been reported that an activating monoclonal antibody directed to the adhesion molecule CD44 markedly reduced the leukemic repopulation of transplanted human AML in NOD-SCID mice, potentially through interference with transport to stem cell-supportive microenvironmental niches and alteration of AML-LSC fate [77].

In addition, a blocking monoclonal antibody against CD47 enabled phagocytosis of ALL cells by macrophages *in vitro* and inhibited tumor engraftment *in vivo* [78]. Significantly, this anti-CD47 antibody eliminated ALL in the peripheral blood, bone marrow, spleen and liver of mice engrafted with primary human ALL, providing preclinical support for such strategy to treathuman ALL [78]. Of particular interest, blockade of CD47 with a monoclonal antibody (mAb) also resulted in macrophage engulfment of human bladder cancer cells *in vitro* and *in vivo* treatment resulted in a significant reduction in the tumor volume of bladder cancer xenografts in a dose-dependent manner [39].

Last, in the search for novel drug discovery platforms, high-throughput screens using small molecules or small interfering RNA (siRNA) libraries have become an area of heated attention [6]. For example, salinomycin has been identified as a compound that dramatically reduces the proportion of breast CSCs, with a >100-fold potency compared to paclitaxel, a commonly used breast cancer chemotherapeutic drug. Importantly, treatment of mice with salinomycin inhibited the mammary tumor growth *in vivo* [79]. Similarly, kinetin riboside (KR) has been identified to specifically eliminate leukemia-initiating cells (LICs) without effecting HSCs [80]. Finally, a genome-wide human kinase siRNA library screen has identified polo-like kinase 1 (PLK1) as critical for breast cancer TIC survival, demonstrating a proof of principle to identify target genes for CSCs [81].

CONCLUSION

In summary, bladder cancer is a heterogeneous disease and much of its notorious malignant behavior, such as drug resistance, tumor recurrence and metastasis, may well be contributed from the roles of bladder cancer stem cells

(CSCs). Therefore, characterization of specific surface markers and identification of dysregulated signaling pathways in bladder CSCs should enlighten us on the better understanding and treatment of this malignancy. It is conceivable that development of novel agents targeting bladder CSCs, on their own or in combination with conventional therapeutics, should greatly benefit bladder cancer patients suffering from both non-invasive and invasive subtypes.

Acknowledgments

This work was supported by Roswell Park Cancer Institute and National Cancer Institute (NCI) grant #P30 CA016056, in part, by the American Cancer Society Institutional Research Grant 02-197-04 and an award from the Roswell Park Alliance Foundation (to J.Z);

References

[1] Castillo-Martin M, Domingo-Domenech J, Karni-Schmidt O, Matos T, & Cordon-Cardo C (2010) Molecular pathways of urothelial development and bladder tumorigenesis. *Urologic oncology* 28(4):401-408.

[2] Goebell PJ & Knowles MA (2010) Bladder cancer or bladder cancers? Genetically distinct malignant conditions of the urothelium. *Urologic oncology* 28(4):409-428.

[3] Zhang CJ, et al., (2012) Engagement of integrinbeta1 induces resistance of bladder cancer cells to mitomycin-C. *Urology* 79(3):638-643.

[4] Bowman KJ, et al., (2014) Comet assay measures of DNA damage are predictive of bladder cancer cell treatment sensitivity in vitro and outcome in vivo. *International journal of cancer. Journal international du cancer* 134(5):1102-1111.

[5] Magee JA, Piskounova E, & Morrison SJ (2012) Cancer stem cells: impact, heterogeneity, and uncertainty. *Cancer cell* 21(3):283-296.

[6] Visvader JE & Lindeman GJ (2012) Cancer stem cells: current status and evolving complexities. *Cell stem cell* 10(6):717-728.

[7] Jordan CT, Guzman ML, & Noble M (2006) Cancer stem cells. *The New England journal of medicine* 355(12):1253-1261.

[8] Holyoake TL, Jiang X, Drummond MW, Eaves AC, & Eaves CJ (2002) Elucidating critical mechanisms of deregulated stem cell turnover in the chronic phase of chronic myeloid leukemia. *Leukemia* 16(4):549-558.

[9] Bonnet D & Dick JE (1997) Human acute myeloid leukemia is organized as a hierarchy that originates from a primitive hematopoietic cell. *Nature medicine* 3(7):730-737.

[10] Castor A, et al., (2005) Distinct patterns of hematopoietic stem cell involvement in acute lymphoblastic leukemia. *Nature medicine* 11(6):630-637.

[11] Eaves CJ, Cashman JD, Zoumbos NC, Barnett MJ, & Eaves AC (1993) Biological strategies for the selective manipulation of normal and leukemic stem cells. *Stem cells* 11 Suppl 3:109-121.

[12] Udomsakdi C, Eaves CJ, Lansdorp PM, & Eaves AC (1992) Phenotypic heterogeneity of primitive leukemic hematopoietic cells in patients with chronic myeloid leukemia. *Blood* 80(10):2522-2530.

[13] Selby P, Bizzari JP, & Buick RN (1983) Therapeutic implications of a stem cell model for human breast cancer: a hypothesis. *Cancer treatment reports* 67(7-8):659-663.

[14] Dontu G, El-Ashry D, & Wicha MS (2004) Breast cancer, stem/progenitor cells and the estrogen receptor. *Trends in endocrinology and metabolism: TEM* 15(5):193-197.

[15] Al-Hajj M, Wicha MS, Benito-Hernandez A, Morrison SJ, & Clarke MF (2003) Prospective identification of tumorigenic breast cancer cells. *Proceedings of the National Academy of Sciences of the United States of America* 100(7):3983-3988.

[16] van Haaften-Day C, et al., (1987) Xenografted small cell undifferentiated cancer of prostate: possible common origin with prostatic adenocarcinoma. *The Prostate* 11(3):271-279.

[17] Jiao J, et al., (2012) Identification of CD166 as a surface marker for enriching prostate stem/progenitor and cancer initiating cells. *PloS one* 7(8):e42564.

[18] Mulholland DJ, et al., (2009) Lin-Sca-1+CD49fhigh stem/progenitors are tumor-initiating cells in the Pten-null prostate cancer model. *Cancer research* 69(22):8555-8562.

[19] Bisson I & Prowse DM (2009) WNT signaling regulates self-renewal and differentiation of prostate cancer cells with stem cell characteristics. *Cell research* 19(6):683-697.

[20] Karhadkar SS, et al., (2004) Hedgehog signalling in prostate regeneration, neoplasia and metastasis. *Nature* 431(7009):707-712.

[21] Leong KG & Gao WQ (2008) The Notch pathway in prostate development and cancer. *Differentiation; research in biological diversity* 76(6):699-716.

[22] Hemmati HD, et al., (2003) Cancerous stem cells can arise from pediatric brain tumors. *Proceedings of the National Academy of Sciences of the United States of America* 100(25):15178-15183.

[23] Kondo T, Setoguchi T, & Taga T (2004) Persistence of a small subpopulation of cancer stem-like cells in the C6 glioma cell line. *Proceedings of the National Academy of Sciences of the United States of America* 101(3):781-786.

[24] Singh SK, et al., (2004) Identification of human brain tumour initiating cells. *Nature* 432(7015):396-401.

[25] Beier D, et al., (2007) CD133(+) and CD133(-) glioblastoma-derived cancer stem cells show differential growth characteristics and molecular profiles. *Cancer research* 67(9):4010-4015.

[26] Wang J, et al., (2008) CD133 negative glioma cells form tumors in nude rats and give rise to CD133 positive cells. *International journal of cancer. Journal international du cancer* 122(4):761-768.

[27] Lathia JD, et al., (2010) Integrin alpha 6 regulates glioblastoma stem cells. *Cell stem cell* 6(5):421-432.

[28] Zhu TS, et al., (2011) Endothelial cells create a stem cell niche in glioblastoma by providing NOTCH ligands that nurture self-renewal of cancer stem-like cells. *Cancer research* 71(18):6061-6072.

[29] McConkey DJ, et al., (2010) Molecular genetics of bladder cancer: Emerging mechanisms of tumor initiation and progression. *Urologic oncology* 28(4):429-440.

[30] Kurzrock EA, Lieu DK, Degraffenried LA, Chan CW, & Isseroff RR (2008) Label-retaining cells of the bladder: candidate urothelial stem cells. *American journal of physiology. Renal physiology* 294(6):F1415-1421.

[31] van der Horst G, Bos L, & van der Pluijm G (2012) Epithelial plasticity, cancer stem cells, and the tumor-supportive stroma in bladder carcinoma. *Molecular cancer research : MCR* 10(8):995-1009.

[32] Crum CP & McKeon FD (2010) p63 in epithelial survival, germ cell surveillance, and neoplasia. *Annual review of pathology* 5:349-371.

[33] Deutsch GB, et al., (2011) DNA damage in oocytes induces a switch of the quality control factor TAp63alpha from dimer to tetramer. *Cell* 144(4):566-576.

[34] Larsson HM, Gorostidi F, Hubbell JA, Barrandon Y, & Frey P (2014) Clonal, self-renewing and differentiating human and porcine urothelial cells, a novel stem cell population. *PloS one* 9(2):e90006.

[35] Pignon JC, et al., (2013) p63-expressing cells are the stem cells of developing prostate, bladder, and colorectal epithelia. *Proceedings of the National Academy of Sciences of the United States of America* 110(20):8105-8110.

[36] Dotsikas G, et al., (1987) Cellular heterogeneity in normal and neoplastic human urothelium: a study using murine monoclonal antibodies. *British journal of cancer* 56(4):439-444.

[37] Cheng L, et al., (2014) Biomarkers in bladder cancer: translational and clinical implications. *Critical reviews in oncology/hematology* 89(1):73-111.

[38] Hatina J & Schulz WA (2012) Stem cells in the biology of normal urothelium and urothelial carcinoma. *Neoplasma* 59(6):728-736.

[39] Chan KS, et al., (2009) Identification, molecular characterization, clinical prognosis, and therapeutic targeting of human bladder tumor-initiating cells. *Proceedings of the National Academy of Sciences of the United States of America* 106(33):14016-14021.

[40] Mhawech-Fauceglia P, Cheney RT, & Schwaller J (2006) Genetic alterations in urothelial bladder carcinoma: an updated review. *Cancer* 106(6):1205-1216.

[41] Koga F, et al., (2003) Impaired p63 expression associates with poor prognosis and uroplakin III expression in invasive urothelial carcinoma of the bladder. *Clinical cancer research : an official journal of the American Association for Cancer Research* 9(15):5501-5507.

[42] Urist MJ, et al., (2002) Loss of p63 expression is associated with tumor progression in bladder cancer. *The American journal of pathology* 161(4):1199-1206.

[43] Koga F, et al., (2003) Impaired Delta Np63 expression associates with reduced beta-catenin and aggressive phenotypes of urothelial neoplasms. *British journal of cancer* 88(5):740-747.

[44] Choi W, et al., (2012) p63 expression defines a lethal subset of muscle-invasive bladder cancers. *PloS one* 7(1):e30206.

[45] Guzman ML, et al., (2001) Nuclear factor-kappaB is constitutively activated in primitive human acute myelogenous leukemia cells. *Blood* 98(8):2301-2307.

[46] Xu Q, Simpson SE, Scialla TJ, Bagg A, & Carroll M (2003) Survival of acute myeloid leukemia cells requires PI3 kinase activation. *Blood* 102(3):972-980.

[47] Wang Y, et al., (2010) The Wnt/beta-catenin pathway is required for the development of leukemia stem cells in AML. *Science* 327(5973):1650-1653.

[48] Dierks C, et al., (2008) Expansion of Bcr-Abl-positive leukemic stem cells is dependent on Hedgehog pathway activation. *Cancer cell* 14(3):238-249.

[49] Zhao C, et al., (2009) Hedgehog signalling is essential for maintenance of cancer stem cells in myeloid leukaemia. *Nature* 458(7239):776-779.

[50] Tan S & Barker N (2014) Epithelial stem cells and intestinal cancer. *Seminars in cancer biology*.

[51] Kinzler KW & Vogelstein B (1996) Lessons from hereditary colorectal cancer. *Cell* 87(2):159-170.

[52] Reya T & Clevers H (2005) Wnt signalling in stem cells and cancer. *Nature* 434(7035):843-850.

[53] Fearon ER & Vogelstein B (1990) A genetic model for colorectal tumorigenesis. *Cell* 61(5):759-767.

[54] Bienz M & Clevers H (2000) Linking colorectal cancer to Wnt signaling. *Cell* 103(2):311-320.

[55] Hiemer SE & Varelas X (2013) Stem cell regulation by the Hippo pathway. *Biochimica et biophysica acta* 1830(2):2323-2334.

[56] Yu FX & Guan KL (2013) The Hippo pathway: regulators and regulations. *Genes & development* 27(4):355-371.

[57] Varelas X, et al., (2008) TAZ controls Smad nucleocytoplasmic shuttling and regulates human embryonic stem-cell self-renewal. *Nature cell biology* 10(7):837-848.

[58] Alarcon C, et al., (2009) Nuclear CDKs drive Smad transcriptional activation and turnover in BMP and TGF-beta pathways. *Cell* 139(4):757-769.

[59] Lian I, et al., (2010) The role of YAP transcription coactivator in regulating stem cell self-renewal and differentiation. *Genes & development* 24(11):1106-1118.

[60] Tamm C, Bower N, & Anneren C (2011) Regulation of mouse embryonic stem cell self-renewal by a Yes-YAP-TEAD2 signaling pathway downstream of LIF. *Journal of cell science* 124(Pt 7):1136-1144.

[61] Camargo FD, et al., (2007) YAP1 increases organ size and expands undifferentiated progenitor cells. *Current biology : CB* 17(23):2054-2060.

[62] Tanaka M, Itoh T, Tanimizu N, & Miyajima A (2011) Liver stem/progenitor cells: their characteristics and regulatory mechanisms. *Journal of biochemistry* 149(3):231-239.

[63] Dong J, et al., (2007) Elucidation of a universal size-control mechanism in Drosophila and mammals. *Cell* 130(6):1120-1133.

[64] Schlegelmilch K, et al., (2011) Yap1 acts downstream of alpha-catenin to control epidermal proliferation. *Cell* 144(5):782-795.

[65] Thiery JP, Acloque H, Huang RY, & Nieto MA (2009) Epithelial-mesenchymal transitions in development and disease. *Cell* 139(5):871-890.

[66] Mani SA, et al., (2008) The epithelial-mesenchymal transition generates cells with properties of stem cells. *Cell* 133(4):704-715.

[67] Overholtzer M, et al., (2006) Transforming properties of YAP, a candidate oncogene on the chromosome 11q22 amplicon. *Proceedings of the National Academy of Sciences of the United States of America* 103(33):12405-12410.

[68] Chan SW, et al., (2008) A role for TAZ in migration, invasion, and tumorigenesis of breast cancer cells. *Cancer research* 68(8):2592-2598.

[69] Cordenonsi M, et al., (2011) The Hippo transducer TAZ confers cancer stem cell-related traits on breast cancer cells. *Cell* 147(4):759-772.

[70] Li X, et al., (2008) Intrinsic resistance of tumorigenic breast cancer cells to chemotherapy. *Journal of the National Cancer Institute* 100(9):672-679.

[71] Bao S, et al., (2006) Glioma stem cells promote radioresistance by preferential activation of the DNA damage response. *Nature* 444(7120):756-760.

[72] Gottesman MM, Fojo T, & Bates SE (2002) Multidrug resistance in cancer: role of ATP-dependent transporters. *Nature reviews. Cancer* 2(1):48-58.

[73] Merchant AA & Matsui W (2010) Targeting Hedgehog--a cancer stem cell pathway. *Clinical cancer research : an official journal of the American Association for Cancer Research* 16(12):3130-3140.

[74] Clement V, Sanchez P, de Tribolet N, Radovanovic I, & Ruiz i Altaba A (2007) HEDGEHOG-GLI1 signaling regulates human glioma growth, cancer stem cell self-renewal, and tumorigenicity. *Current biology : CB* 17(2):165-172.

[75] Bar EE, et al., (2007) Cyclopamine-mediated hedgehog pathway inhibition depletes stem-like cancer cells in glioblastoma. *Stem cells* 25(10):2524-2533.

[76] Liu S, et al., (2006) Hedgehog signaling and Bmi-1 regulate self-renewal of normal and malignant human mammary stem cells. *Cancer research* 66(12):6063-6071.

[77] Jin L, Hope KJ, Zhai Q, Smadja-Joffe F, & Dick JE (2006) Targeting of CD44 eradicates human acute myeloid leukemic stem cells. *Nature medicine* 12(10):1167-1174.

[78] Chao MP, et al., (2011) Therapeutic antibody targeting of CD47 eliminates human acute lymphoblastic leukemia. *Cancer research* 71(4):1374-1384.

[79] Gupta PB, et al., (2009) Identification of selective inhibitors of cancer stem cells by high-throughput screening. *Cell* 138(4):645-659.

[80] McDermott SP, et al., (2012) A small molecule screening strategy with validation on human leukemia stem cells uncovers the therapeutic efficacy of kinetin riboside. *Blood* 119(5):1200-1207.

[81] Hu K, Law JH, Fotovati A, & Dunn SE (2012) Small interfering RNA library screen identified polo-like kinase-1 (PLK1) as a potential therapeutic target for breast cancer that uniquely eliminates tumor-initiating cells. *Breast cancer research : BCR* 14(1):R22.

In: Bladder Cancer
Editor: Samantha Haggerty

ISBN: 978-1-63321-666-2

Chapter 2

THE FIVE SENSES IN BLADDER CANCER DIAGNOSTICS

Caterina Gulia[1], Giacinto Marrocco[2], Santiago Vallasciani[3] and Roberto Piergentili[4*]

[1]Dipartimento di Scienze Ginecologico-Ostetriche e Scienze Urologiche, Policlinico Umberto I, Sapienza - Università di Roma, Italia
[2]UOC di Chirurgia ed Urologia Pediatrica, Azienda Ospedaliera San Camillo-Forlanini, Roma, Italia
[3]UOSD di Urologia Pediatrica, Policlinico Maggiore, Milano, Italia
[4]Istituto di Biologia, Medicina Molecolare e Nanobiotecnologie del CNR; Dipartimento di Biologia e Biotecnologie, Sapienza - Università di Roma, Italia

ABSTRACT

Bladder carcinoma (BC) is the second most common malignancy of the urinary tract in males after prostate cancer. Diagnosis is usually subsequent to patients' report of blood in the urine (macrohematuria) frequently without pain. Yet, macrohematuria may be also associated to other bladder conditions such as stones, infections, or benign tumors, and its presence may be intermittent or not assessable without a specific test (urinalysis), thus bleeding is sometimes diagnosed serendipitously during routine checkups. Bleeding in BC is caused by the presence of fragile

* Corresponding Author: RP – roberto.piergentili@uniroma1.it.

tissue, but this is related neither to the stage nor to the extension of the neoplastic lesion. Other non-exclusive symptoms involve irritative bladder behaviors, such as changes in urination frequency, dysuria and urgency; in case of large cancers, lower back pain or inability to urinate may be present. Also in these situations, the abovementioned symptoms may be associated to other clinical conditions not related to BC. Thus, it is extremely important to verify its presence and to perform an accurate differential diagnosis. *Hearing* the patient, and accurately report all symptoms and possible risk factors during anamnesis (smoking, professional exposure to chemicals, persistent phlogosis) is thus crucial to address him/her to a specialist for more specific analyses. A reliable assessment of BC presence and stage may be obtained mainly by a *visual*, direct analysis of the bladder followed by subsequent evaluation of a specialist urologist, using cystoscopy, tomography, ultrasonography and urinary cytology. These techniques will be analyzed here and newest frontiers in their development will be explained. We will show an overview of the most used biological markers of BC traceable inside urine and used for both diagnosis and stadiation purposes, allowing to *taste* urine content and helping in both diagnosis and possible cure. We will illustrate the mechanism of action of a palpation device, that allows differentiating normal and cancer samples by *touching* a bioptic specimen. We will also describe a recently developed technique able to *smell* volatile molecules from the urine of patients and to help in diagnosis. Finally, we will describe recent advances in BC diagnostics obtained by electrical impedance spectroscopy.

INTRODUCTION

According to the US National Cancer Institute (NCI) website (accession: April 2014) (http://www.cancer.gov) bladder cancer (BC) is classified among the most common cancer types in the USA. Estimations for year 2014 in this country account for almost 75,000 new cases, and more than 15,000 deaths. In 2013, about 55,000 men and 18,000 women had been diagnosed with bladder cancer in the United States, with a ratio of approximately 3:1. Consequently, in this country BC is the sixth cause of cancer as for new cases, and the eighth cause of death among common cancers. As for urogenital neoplasms, BC is second only to prostate cancer in males and has an incidence higher than kidney cancers (including both renal cells and renal pelvis). The United States SEER (Surveillance, Epidemiology, and End Results) Program reports that in 2013 BC accounted for 4.4% of all new cancer cases and was responsible of 2.6% of all cancer deaths. In 2010, prevalence data accounted for more than

560,000 people having BC in the USA only, with a lifetime risk of ca. 2.4%. SEER data during the time frame 2003-2009 show that survival at 5 years is less than 78%. As expected, an early diagnosis is strictly related to higher 5-years survival rate, with in situ BC accounting for 96.4%; instead, if BC metastasized, survival is as low as 5.4%. BC is a typical age-related disease - more than 70% of affected patients are 65 years old or elder, with a peak at age frame 75-84 (>30%), and a median age at diagnosis of 73 years. The medical cost related to BC treatment - due to patients' treatment, surveillance protocols, recurrence rates - had been extensively studied over the time (Botteman et al., 2003; Sievert et al., 2009; Svatek et al., 2014). Mariotto and collaborators (Mariotto et al., 2011) estimate that in the US, the direct cost for this disease was 125 billions in 2010 only, with an expected increase up to 155 billion by year 2020. Complications significantly contribute to the life-time costs of managing bladder cancer (Avritscher et al., 2006), thus it becomes crucial, both for the health of the patients and for the cost for society, to diagnose BC as early and as precisely as possible. The well known golden rule is that a precocious therapy, subsequent to an early diagnosis, significantly increases patients life quality and decreases both recurrences and surveillance related costs. In this perspective, being able to recognize this disease in the very early steps of its development is, consequently, a priority.

HEARING BC: THE IMPORTANCE OF AN ACCURATE ANAMNESIS

BC, especially in its early steps, may be a non-painful condition, and the only clue about a bladder problem is often patient's report of an abnormally colored urine (Table 1) (West, 2013). In these cases, the presence of a bleeding lesion inside this organ may be hypothesized only in the presence of reddish urine, caused by macrohematuria. Yet, this symptom in BC affected patients may be intermittent, of variable entity (different red tones according to blood quantity) or even completely absent; indeed, only 4% to 10% of BC patients reports this symptom (Grossfeld and Carroll, 1998). To further complicate this scenario, macrohematuria may be also related to all medical conditions causing lesions in the urogenital apparatus, including (but not limited to) kidney and/or bladder stones, urinary tract infections, mechanical lesions during work or sport activities, and so on. Then, it is crucial to correctly address all possible aspects of patient's life, in order to find possible risk factors involved in BC formation.

Table 1. Urine colors and their relation with medical conditions, according to West (West, 2013)

urine color	dye	most common cause	related disease(s)
red	blood	lesions in the urogenital tract	bladder cancer, kidney or bladder stones, infections, benign tumors
pink	beet juice	diet	none
orange	phenazopyridine, urinary tract antibiotics, carotene	drug administration; diet	urinary tract infection
dark brown / black	bilirubine	excess bilirubine production	liver cancer
dark yellow	urobilin	dehydratation	no
pale yellow	urobilin	hyperhydratation	no
cloudy yellow	bacteria	urinary infection	urinary tract infection
blue	drugs (viagra, indomethacin, propofol); chemicals (methylene blue); food dyes	medical treatments; diet	carbon monoxide poisoning and malaria treatment; surgery
green	drugs; chemicals; dies; urinary tract infection	a diluted blue urine; bacterial infection	as above
indigo / violet / purple	blood; porphyrins; heme	purple urine bag syndrome (urinary tract infection and highly alkaline urine); porphyria	kidney failure; porphyria

Tobacco smoking, either active or passive, is the most well established risk factor for BC in both sexes (Pelucchi et al., 2006; Murta-Nascimento et al., 2007; Letasiova et al., 2012). Smoking is directly related to both duration of smoking habits and quantity of cigarettes per day; moreover, also tabagism starting age is an important risk factor: people who started at younger ages are more prone to develop BC, even if both previously mentioned parameters have the same values (Freedman et al., 2011; Yang, 2011; Ferris et al., 2013).

Occupational exposure is another risk factor in BC epidemiology. Connected to the smoke, the risk for fire fighters is described in literature (Golka and Weistenhöfer, 2008). Combustion of substances such as polymers (foams based on polyurethanes), paints and coatings, during thermal degradation may release chemicals - aromatic amines, polycyclic aromatic hydrocarbons - directly related to urogenital cancer formation. In the list of chemicals connected to BC formation is also possible to include aniline dyes, nitrites and nitrates (Messing, 2004). Aromatic amines, likely the most studied compounds involved in this disease, are also found in industrial processes of firms producing chemicals (such as fungicides), dyes (for example, paints), rubber and plastics; also metal and motor vehicle exhaust and pollutant emissions from industrial installations had been connected to BC formation (Garcia-Perez et al., 2009; Letasiova et al., 2012). In this perspective, it is important not only to verify patients' job, but also if their houses are in close proximity of such industries. Interestingly, some amines are also present in hair dyes. Although literature reports either significant (Gago-Dominguez et al., 2001) or not significant at all (Ros et al., 2012) the risk increase for personal use of these dyes, there is an increased and statistically significant risk of BC among hairdressers (Harling et al., 2010), this suggesting a dose- and time of exposure-dependent role of these molecules in the disease.

Another possible risk factor is the dietary habit of the patient (Ferris et al., 2013), possibly connected to his/her geographical origin or usual living place. The presence of arsenic and/or chromium chlorination byproducts in the food chain - especially drinking water, but also grains, vegetables, meats, fish, or food processed with arsenic-containing water - had been repeatedly related to BC formation (Ferris et al., 2013; Oberoi et al., 2014). Although the exact relationship between arsenic and this neoplasm is not fully understood, several evidences accumulated in the last years about a possible epigenetic role of this substance in promoting aberrant gene expression through DNA hyper- or hypo-methylation (Bustaffa et al., 2014). Interestingly, however, drinking lots of (arsenic-free) water significantly decreases the risk of developing BC (Lotan et al., 2013). It is likely that this effect is due to the consequent frequent urination, which keeps chemicals from lingering in the body. In addition, other naturally occurring chemicals may be involved in BC formation; in particular, evidences exist about the role that excess copper, or iron and zinc deficiency, play in the disease (Mazdak et al., 2010). Instead and surprisingly, excess alcohol drinking failed to be unequivocally associated to this cancer, independently of both quality and quantity (Mao et al., 2010; Pelucchi et al., 2012). Similarly, also milk consumption seems unrelated to BC formation (Mao et al., 2011), this being surprising since this beverage is indeed connected to both ovarian (Larsson et al., 2006) and prostate (Qin et al., 2007) cancer formation.

Type 2 diabetes patients may be at risk of higher incidence of BC (Gallagher and LeRoith, 2013), also depending on the therapy they use to lower the levels of circulating glucose. Data available from literature show that some of these compounds might be involved in BC formation. Thiazolidinediones (TZDs) are a class of oral glucose-lowering drugs whose function is to increase insulin sensitivity and insulin resistance. To date, three compounds have ever been approved for human use: troglitazone, rosiglitazone, and pioglitazone. The first two were subsequently withdrawn from the market because of side effects. Pioglitazone is still in the market, but there are evidences that this molecule may increase BC risk (Tseng, 2014).

Chronic urinary tract infections are also directly related to BC development. It has been reported that molecules mediating immune response - such as interleukin-2 (IL-2) (Shen et al., 2012) and, possibly, IL-4, IL-4R and IL-13 (Chu et al., 2012) - are involved in the development of this cancer. Thus, infections that chronically affect some populations would be able to promote BC formation as well. This has been repeatedly reported for schistosomiasis (bilharzia) which has been considered a definitive cause of urinary bladder cancer with an associated five-fold risk (Mostafa et al., 1999; Alibek et al., 2012), especially where this infection is endemic, such as Egypt (Bedwani et al., 1998). Virus infections may as well be strongly correlated to BC formation, as demonstrated for human papilloma virus (HPV) (Alibek et al., 2012), especially for the HPV16 and HPV18 forms (Frank et al., 2002). Also polyomavirus JCV seems to be associated to BC (Shen et al., 2011), thus the geographical origin of the patient or a recent, even transient, transfer in some risky countries may, again, play an important role in BC etiology.

As expected, BC may also be a consequence of the therapy of another neoplasm, or a relapse/recurrence of a formerly treated BC. External beam radiation therapy (EBRT) for urogenital malignancies increases the rate of secondary bladder cancer formation, thus a careful follow-up in patients undergoing ERBT or similar therapies should be performed, particularly in young patients (Nieder et al., 2008). The use of cyclophosphamide, an alkylating agent used in chemotherapy, has been correlated with later development of muscle-invasive bladder cancer (MIBC), with a latency of 6-

13 years. Similarly, acrolein, a metabolite of cyclophosphamide, used in the treatment of some tumors such as non-Hodgkin's lymphoma, is responsible for the increase in the incidence of BC (Kaldor et al., 1995; Travis et al., 1995). In the last years, several new molecules had been tested or are under clinical trial for BC cure (Piergentili et al., 2014), but for most of them long-term effect on BC relapse and/or recurrence is still unknown. Hence, a previous patient's history of cancer treatment (even if not a BC) is an important point to keep in mind during anamnesis.

BC may also be connected with developmental anomalies during gestation. For example, if the urachus persists after birth, it may originate adenocarcinomas; it is estimated that approximately one third of all bladder adenocarcinomas (which are, in any case, a minority of the BCs, counting approximately 1% of all cases) have this origin. In these patients, sometimes hematuria is accompanied by mucosuria (Ogaya Piniés et al., 2012). This type of BC affects almost exclusively adults, and pediatric cases are extremely rare (Gupta et al., 2014 and references therein). Another cause of bladder adenocarcinoma is bladder exstrophy (Roy and Parwani, 2011). In this pathology, both the bladder and the abdominal wall facing it fail to close completely during development and, instead, are fused together, thus leaving the inner bladder wall exposed to the external environment. Although surgically corrected, this leaves the patient with a predisposition to both urinary tract infections and BC.

Quite an high number of additional risk factors had been identified, regarding the socio-economic and/or the physiological state of the patient, which hence should be considered during anamnesis. Age and gender quantitative influences are highlighted in the Introduction. Yet, as for the gender role in the disease, some additional considerations had been investigated in the literature. Available data reveal that BC staging T1 to T3 affects both sexes equally as for survival, but a difference is evident for stage T4a (May et al., 2011). Convincing explanations of these data are still under investigation, though some physiological variables (such as anatomical and/or hormonal differences) are discussed in literature (Shariat et al., 2010; Scosyrev et al., 2010). Socio-economic considerations may be also considered when describing differential race-related BC incidence and survival. It is generally accepted that black people have a poorer survival compared to white people; this fact is usually connected to higher BC stage at presentation (Lee et al., 2006; Yee et al., 2011). However, these difference persists if similarly staged patients are compared (Underwood et al., 2006). Some Authors (Yee et al., 2011) hypothesize that these discrepancies may be at least partially ascribed to differential quality of treatment, access to and quality of care, surveillance after primary treatment, and comorbidity. Finally, some scientists also think that even marital status might be taken into account, when evaluating cancer survival (Gore at al., 2005), probably because of the major awareness of women for their health and, consequently, for that of their husbands.

Lastly, BC may also occur because of a genetic predisposition; in this case, quite an high number of genes had been identified, which are either mutated or erroneously regulated in BC cells (Di Pierro et al., 2012). Remembering to ask the patients about other cases of cancer in their family, and not just BC, is then very important: the two pivotal genes in this condition are TP53 and FGFR3, which are either mutated or deregulated also in many other neoplasms (see http://omim.org/entry/191170 for TP53 and http://omim.org/entry/134934 for FGFR3).

VIEWING BC: INNOVATIVE APPROACHES IN IMAGING DIAGNOSTICS

After anamnesis, the physician may decide to send the patient to the urologist to verify the presence of a bladder lesion and, in positive cases, evaluate its entity and extension. In this field, imaging techniques are usually the first and most important step to assess the presence of a BC. Imaging techniques may include different approaches, and the most used techniques are ultrasonography (US), cystoscopy, tomography (CT), and magnetic resonance (NMR). Ultrasonography is the easiest way to analyze a bladder, but its efficiency in BC diagnostics is mainly limited to superficial lesions (Hafeez and Huddart, 2013), despite technical improvements such as two- and three-dimensional trans-abdominal ultrasound. An even more improved US technique, namely three-dimensional contrast-enhanced ultrasound, had been recently developed, and it is reported as able to discriminate between muscle invasive (MIBC) and non-invasive (NMIBC) bladder cancers (Li et al., 2012); however its use is not yet widespread, and consequently its real value is still under investigation for both sensitivity and specificity.

Compared to ultrasonography, cystoscopy is invasive, time-consuming and expensive. It consists of inserting a live imaging device - a microscopic camera based on optic fiber technology, equipped with a white light source - inside a special tube (cystoscope) and the tube through the urethra. To date, cystoscopy is the most affordable and used way of investigation. The specialist may also decide to take a sample of the bladder tissue for further analysis (biopsy) using the same device to perform a transurethral resection (TUR). Although regional anesthesia is usually adopted during cystoscopy, TUR normally requires a total one. The cystoscope may also be used to resect a BC (transurethral resection of bladder tumor, or TURBT); also in this case, of course, a total anesthesia is mandatory. Cystoscopy performed with visible light may be improved by narrow band imaging (NBI) (Herr, 2011), which is basically a filter able to detect a special blue/green wavelength inside white light, thus allowing to perform both analyses at the same time (Chen et al., 2013). NBI permits to evaluate the penetration of the beam inside bladder walls, thus enhancing the contrast between blood vessels and surrounding tissue, highlighting structural differences between normal and transformed tissue. A variant of visible light cystoscopy is the photodynamic diagnosis (PDD), or "blue-light cystoscopy" (Lerner et al., 2012). In this analysis the urologist first injects a drug - either 5-aminolevulinic acid (5-ALA) or its derivate hexyl-aminolevulinate (HAL) - which is specifically adsorbed by cancer cells (Oude Elferink and Witjes, 2014); in this way, instead of normal white light, the specialist will use a special blue light which will make cancer cells glow by fluorescence, thus increasing diagnostic accuracy in respect to white light cystoscopy only (Lapini et al., 2012). Although PDD is quite safe and well tolerated, it has some important drawbacks, such as relatively low specificity and elevated costs (Cordeiro et al., 2013). A further improvement in this field is the three-dimensional optical coherence tomography (3D-OCT) with quantitative computer aided detection. This technique significantly improves the sensitivity of both white light cystoscopy and fluorescence cystoscopy, and the specificity of NBI for early diagnosis for flat and early lesions, such as initial carcinoma *in situ* (CIS) (Ren et al., 2012). In any case, the definitive diagnosis of bladder cancer requires histopathological confirmation. Thus, the direct analysis of the cystoscopic specimen is still a necessary, subsequent step in suspect cases. Cytology may be also performed on urine samples, by analyzing floating material in search of neoplastic cells; this technique is far less invasive than cystoscopy, and it may be coupled with the search of cancer molecular markers (see next section).

More complex imaging techniques involve computerized tomography (CT) and nuclear magnetic resonance (NMR), but they require very expensive equipment and for this they are used only in specialized centers. During CT, a computerized tomograph takes a series of X-rays scans and then the computer merges them to obtain a three-dimensional image of the bladder; the use of a contrast dye - either drinkable or injectable - is not mandatory. The 64-slice

CT has both an high sensitivity (85%) and specificity (94%) in BC diagnostics (Martingano et al., 2010), but both morphology (flat lesions, carcinoma *in situ*) and size (<1cm) of bladder lesions may impair a correct evaluation of the disease. Moreover, the operator experience is important as well in diagnosing a BC, and the technique fails to correctly discriminate among bladder layers (MacVicar, 2000; Tritschler et al., 2012).

The computerized tomography may also be coupled with a positron emission tomography (PET) during the same diagnostic session. In this case, it is possible to investigate functional - and not merely morphological - tissue alterations, in search of a neoplastic formation. Thus, composite PET/CT scans may provide both molecular and histological information regarding bladder status. The dye is chosen according to the wanted investigation; ^{18}F-fludeoxyglucose (18-FDG) is generically used to visualize cancer cells because of their increased glucose metabolism, and this marker is able to detect neoplastic cells even before any morphological tissue/organ change, thus allowing PET/CT to outperform both CT and NMR in very early BC stages (Antoch et al., 2004). However, this technique shows some weaknesses. First, it measures augmented glucose consumption without discriminate the cause of this increase; thus, phlogosis, infection or increased individual metabolism might all be scored as false positives (Saksena, 2006). Second, the bladder-mediated excretion of the isotope may create artificial accumulations inside the organ, thus generating additional false positives (Harkirat et al., 2010). Third, its sensitivity dramatically drops when evaluating BC recurrence after a preceding chemotherapy (Liu et al., 2006). In the last years some centers switched from 18-FDG to ^{11}C-choline, a marker of cell membranes whose turnover is increased in cancer cells. The advantages of this dye is given by (i) its low uptake inside normal bladders (de Jong et al., 2002) thus allowing to visualize BC, and (ii) the possibility to evaluate lymph node involvement (Gofrit et al., 2006).

An NMR scan is similar to a CT scan, but it takes advantage of strong magnets and radio waves instead of X-rays to create high-resolution pictures. It is superior to other techniques because of high soft tissue resolution, multiplanar capacity and the possibility to enhance picture contrast using different sequences of images. NMR, especially the functional scans, come in several different "flavors", each having both pros and cons. For some of these scans, a contrast dye may be injected. However, the use of gadolinium-containing dyes should be avoided in all patients with impaired renal function (Thomsen, 2009). An enhancement of standard NMR is the dynamic contrast-enhanced (DCE) NMR; in this case it is possible to visualize *in vivo* the blood flux throughout the entire bladder, to verify the presence of hypoxic areas, typical of BC regions (Padhani and Husband, 2001; Tuncbilek et al., 2009). The analysis of differential aerobic status of bladder tissues is also obtained by blood-oxygenation-level-dependent (BOLD) NMR; contrarily to DCE-NMR,where a paramagnetic contrast agent is required, the only treatment the patient needs to perform is inhaling high oxygen concentrations prior to scanning (Taylor et al., 2001). Instead, diffusion-weighted (DW) NMR is able to discriminate cell concentration by measuring water molecules mobility, and thus identifying the higher cellular numerosity of BC compared to the surrounding, normal tissue (Takeuchi et al., 2009; Kobayashi et al., 2011). The invasiveness of BC may be evaluated by nanoparticle-enhanced (NE) NMR. In this case, lymph node involvement may be investigated by injecting in vein lymphotropic nanoparticles which will be cleared in normal nodes but not in those containing malignant tissues (Thoeny et al., 2009). More recently, there had been attempts to couple PET and DW-NMR (Pichler et al., 2010); although the advantage - in terms of time spent for test execution - is quite evident if paralleled to PET/CT (parallel the former, sequential the latter), the technique is not yet sufficiently used and widespread to evaluate if it is also significantly more effective as a diagnostic tool for BC, compared to straight functional NMRs.

We conclude this section briefly describing an innovative diagnostic approach, which is still in test phase: photoacoustic (PA) imaging (Zackrisson et al., 2014). It is based on the photoacoustic effect: in simple words, a red-light laser beam hits a tissue and the photons heat locally the organ, causing a thermal expansion (thermoelastic effect). The expansion causes pressure waves which can be detected by broadband ultrasonic transducers and converted into images. In humans, the technique had been tested mainly on breast cancers (Zackrisson et al., 2014), but some studies performed on animal bladders anticipate that PA is useful also to determine microvascular differences between malignant and benign bladder tissues without using harmful dyes; animals used so far include dogs (Xie et al., 2011), rats (Jeon et al., 2013) and pigs (Kamaya et al., 2013).

TASTING BC: THE ANALYSIS OF URINE CONTENT

The attempt to guess a disease by tasting urine samples is very old and, historically, the first disease identified in this way is diabetes mellitus (Peumery, 1987). The papyrus from Eberes (1552 B.C.) suggests that

Egyptians were already aware of a disease associated to increased urination. In an ancient Indian document (400 B.C.) Suhsruta Samhita describes a honey-tasting urine (*madhumeda*). In Europe this fact was officially rediscovered by Thomas Willis in 1674, as described in his book *Pharmaceutice Rationalis*. Indeed, urine samples alteration is frequently associated to altered metabolism and disease (Table 1), thus it is conceivable to use it as a diagnostic tool in BC.

At the cellular level, it is possible to retrieve, inside the urine, exfoliation cells coming from bladder internal walls. This analysis, called urine cytology, permits to identify, among the others, the presence of cancer or pre-cancer cells; the test is *per se* not very good for diagnosis if not coupled with other analyses such as cystoscopy, since false negatives are quite frequent. In many cases urine cytology is performed together with urine culture to investigate the presence of urinary tract infections and permitting a differential diagnosis in case of non-specific symptoms. An attempt to improve reliability of this test is the use of fluorescent *in situ* hybridization (FISH) for the evaluation of the presence of additional chromosomes, since genomic instabilities and aneuploidies have been found in BC bioptic samples, mainly involving chromosomes 1, 3, 7, 9, 11 and 17; results indeed improved, yet false signals and sample heterogeneity are still issues (Ke et al., 2014). In this context, an attempt to (at least partially) automatize FISH is UroVysion™ Bladder Cancer Kit, an FDA-approved kit optimized for identifying and quantitating chromosomes 3, 7, 17, and locus 9p21 in human urine specimens. However, as the producer itself states in the related web page, two facts should be taken into account when using it: (i) possible presence of false negatives, since some bladder cancers show genetic changes not detected by the FISH test; (ii) Ta stage solitary tumors smaller than 5mm could not be detected since FISH results rely on the quantity of tumor cells recovered during the process. Consequently, the test is optimized towards identification of high grade BC and, in those cases, fails to show a significant improvement over standard cytology (Moonen et al., 2007).

To date, tests analyzing molecular markers connected to BC formation are far more reliable than urine cytology. The advantage of this approach is that it is minimally invasive, but results obtained so far are not yet completely convincing. Potentially, several proteins may be identified, released in the urine either because of BC metabolism or as a consequence of apoptotic/necrotic cell death consequent to malignancy. For example, the basic fibroblast growth factor (bFGF), a protein with pro-angiogenic activity (Chodak et al., 1988), increases its urine concentration with more advanced stages of the disease (Shariat et al., 2010); however, the relationship between bFGF and BC is not biunivocal, thus potentially leading to erroneous diagnoses. Several other peptides are under evaluation, however the reported panel of molecules may be not highly specific (Schiffer et al., 2009; Chen et al., 2012). By coupling urine cytology and gene expression, some Authors discovered that in the urine it is possible to evaluate the methylation of specific genes and their mis-expression by comparing samples from controls and BC patients. In this way, some protein markers are quite promising. Endothelin receptor type B (EDNRB), APC (adenomatous polyposis coli), TERT_a and TERT_b (telomerase subunits), are part of a panel of markers able to discriminate between tumors and controls using voided urine (Zuiverloon et al., 2012). In the same way, other groups identified additional promising proteins; here we remember GDF15 (growth differentiation factor 15, involved in apoptosis), TMEFF2 (tomoregulin-2, important for cell survival), VIM (Vimentin, a type III intermediate filament) (Costa et al., 2010), ZNF154 (a zinc finger protein coding gene), POU4F2 (a transcription factor), HOXA9 (a homeobox motif containing protein), EOMES (eomesodermin, containing a DNA binding domain) (Reinert et al., 2011). Recent advances in the field include in the list also FGFR3, a tyrosine kinase receptor implicated in cell cycle control and angiogenesis. FGFR3 improper activation - either by mutations in the coding sequence or by alterations in its regulatory pathways - is present in 60% of BC samples (Gomez-Roman et al., 2005; Mhawech-Fauceglia et al., 2007). A recent report shows that this gene may be a good candidate target for BC surveillance of patients treated for non-muscle invasive urothelial carcinoma, as traced in urine specimens (van Kessel et al., 2013).

Alternatively, urine samples may be also tested for the presence of micro-RNA (miR) connected to BC formation and/or development. The list of BC-related miR is relatively long (Di Pierro et al., 2012) and is still increasing in size (Tölle et al., 2013; Mlcochova et al., 2014; Shi et al., 2014). The same analysis may also be related to BC staging; it has been reported that, although with some exceptions, miR down-regulation is typical of low-grade BC, while up-regulation is more common in high-grade cancers (Catto et al., 2009). Notably, also miR expression profile between low and high grade BC is different, suggesting that some of them are directly involved in BC formation and that they may have different effects, likely because they target distinct mRNA (Veerla et al., 2009; Catto et al., 2010).

Another pioneer approach is the use of *metabonomics*, that is the search inside urine of metabolites potentially useful as cancer biomarkers and not directly related to any genotype, expression profile, or even proteome (Holmes et al., 2008; Spratlin et al., 2009). For example, evidences exist that carnitine C9:1 and component-I might be highly specific and prognostic of BC presence and development (Huang et al., 2011).

In an attempt to search BC molecular markers in other body fluids, Osman and collaborators reported the use of blood cell-derived RNA for this purpose (Osman et al., 2006). In their study, they show that blood cells gene expression signatures can discriminate between patients with BC and healthy controls, and among patients with other types of urogenital tumors. Specifically, speaking of BC, they identified seven genes; of them, four (*IGFBP7, SNX16, CSPG6, CTSD*) are overexpressed, and three (*CHD2, NELL2, TNFRSF7*) are underexpressed in BC patients, compared to controls. However, the mechanisms causing differential gene expression in circulating blood cells of BC patients and controls is still unknown and under investigation.

Touching BC: The Use of a "Palpation Device" to Test Tumor Stiffness

In 2011 Lee and collaborators developed a specific palpation device able to "measure tissue behavior against an indentation and estimate the mechanical property (elasticity) of tissues" (Lee et al., 2011). The rationale for this research is to reduce patients' stress upon surgical intervention (partial cystectomy). A way to obtain this, is to reduce as much as possible the size of the removed tissue. However, to obtain that, it is necessary to exactly know neoplasm localization and identify with high precision its margins, especially when trying to individuate intravesical cancer borders from the external wall of the bladder. The machine was tested on explanted samples from patients within 30 minutes from surgery and before histopathology. Resistance of the tissue was measured by a 3 mm indentation (rate: 1 mm/sec) using a force transducer, and the test was repeated several times per each sample, in different areas of the specimen. Both force and tissue deformation were recorded and analyzed; in particular, four BC samples were measured 43 times, and for the controls the Authors used surrounding areas devoid of visible cancerous tissue. BC specimens derived from one woman and three men (mean age: 58.8; range: 44-74) were evaluated. The measured mean elastic modulus was significantly different (BC tissue being stiffer) between healthy and morbid tissue, with a p value of 0.003. The machine is surely interesting, although this technology is still in its infancy, at least for BC evaluation. However, this is for sure a pioneering work in the field of BC elastographic study. If appropriately developed, potentially it should permit to pinpoint the exact extension of the neoplastic lesion in a hassle-free way and, as also underlined in the manuscript, to resolve the problem of the absence of haptic feedback in robotics. It should be remembered, though, that described preliminary tests were performed in a laboratory and after surgery; the ideal situation would be to integrate the palpation device inside a cystoscope or a similar gear, and to further test it *in vivo*, since in this situation the tissue might have slightly yet significantly different elastic characteristics.

SMELLING BC: IN SEARCH OF URINE VOLATILE MOLECULES

In year 2004 the British Medical Journal reported the successful attempt of some scientists to train a group of dogs in identifying BC patients by smelling their urine (Willis et al., 2004). The study showed that dogs indeed had the ability to recognize a characteristic bladder cancer odor, and that this smell was independent of other chemical aspects of the urine detectable by urinalysis. The most recent advance in this field is the so-called "Odoreader" (as some newspapers and televisions called it), basically a GC-sensor device able to capture and analyze volatiles from urine headspace (Khalid et al., 2013). Volatile organic compounds (VOCs) are captured by a conventional gas chromatography (GC) oven fitted with a commercially available capillary column interfaced to a heated metal oxide sensor used as the detector. The comparison of chromatograms from BC patients and controls revealed a typical peak at 3200 (half seconds) which was present in 20/24 bladder cancer samples but absent from controls, and an overall chromatographic profile always and significantly different from that of healthy patients. The molecular identification of VOCs is not investigated in the manuscript, but it likely reflects the altered metabolism of neoplastic cells. Statistically, obtained results are equal or better than currently available urinary biomarkers for bladder cancer, with a prediction value >95% in BC-derived urine samples. Additionally, the device is of low cost, easy to use and with a high lifetime (possibly more than 100 analyses), making it highly promising in BC near-future diagnostics.

Additional Diagnostic Approaches: Identifying BC by Electric Impedance

The increased electric impedance of BC samples, both *ex vivo* and *in vivo*, is a well known fact: the impedivity of the malignant bladder tissue is significantly ($p < 0.001$) higher than that of the benign tissue, especially at lower frequencies (Keshtkar et al., 2006). The reason of this circumstance is quite clear: BC malignant cells are not only metabolically different from their normal counterparts, but show a number of morphological alterations, including (i) larger nuclei, (ii) variable cellular dimensions, shape and orientation, (iii) changes in overall tissue stiffness (see also above) due to impaired cell cohesion (Ro et al., 1992); all these parameters are able to influence the transmission of an electric signal inside a tissue. Thus, the electrical impedance spectroscopy *in vivo* basically consists in inserting two electrodes inside the body and measuring the resulting potential. To make this test even less invasive, it has been subsequently tailored for single cells measurements, using a dielectrophoresis (DEP) microchip with microcavity array and multilayer electrodes (Chuang et al., 2009). The Authors found that the impedance of higher-grade (IV) BC cells was smaller than that of lower-grade (II) BC cells, and the impedance of normal bladder cell was much higher than the values of both cancer cell types. Recently, the system has been further improved from a technical point of view (Chuang et al., 2011) by integrating a PC-based LabVIEW program in the DEP chip. Therefore, the Authors created the bases to produce industrially a system-level biochip for cell analysis on a microchip in the next future. In theory, it should even be possible to envisage the opportunity to couple such a device with other above-mentioned techniques (such as urine cytology) and to couple it with other diagnostic tools to further improve analytic reliability of otherwise less affordable tools such as the UroVysion™ kit.

Conclusion

BC is a widespread pathology potentially caused by a large number of different and frequently unrelated causes. For many characteristics, BC is not really different from other tumors: it shares both genetic (TP53) and non-genetic (smoke, air pollution) causes with other malignancies. Prevention should be a priority in its management, yet the high number of variables to take into account makes it hard to perform. Then, it is crucial to develop either new investigation techniques, or to improve existing ones, to obtain an accurate and precocious diagnosis. To date, there is not just one kind of test that gives certainty to discriminate healthy and morbid bladders, and false positives and negatives are still an issue. At the moment, the recommendation is thus to perform more than one check, possibly using unrelated (i.e., different "senses") techniques.

REFERENCES

Alibek K; Karatayeva N; Bekniyazov I. The role of infectious agents in urogenital cancers. *Infect Agent Cancer.* 2012 Dec 3;7(1):35. doi: 10.1186/1750-9378-7-35.

Antoch G; Saoudi N; Kuehl H; Dahmen G; Mueller SP; Beyer T; Bockisch A; Debatin JF; Freudenberg LS. Accuracy of whole-body dual-modality fluorine-18-2-fluoro-2-deoxy-D-glucose positron emission tomography and computed tomography (FDG-PET/CT) for tumor staging in solid tumors: comparison with CT and PET. *J. Clin. Oncol.* 2004 Nov 1;22(21):4357-68.

Avritscher EB; Cooksley CD; Grossman HB; Sabichi AL; Hamblin L; Dinney CP; Elting LS. Clinical model of lifetime cost of treating bladder cancer and associated complications. *Urology.* 2006 Sep;68(3):549-53.

Bedwani R; Renganathan E; El Kwhsky F; Braga C; Abu Seif HH; Abul Azm T; Zaki A; Franceschi S; Boffetta P; La Vecchia C. Schistosomiasis and the risk of bladder cancer in Alexandria, Egypt. *Br. J. Cancer.* 1998 Apr;77(7):1186-9.

Botteman, MF; Pashos, CL; Redaelli, A; Laskin, B; Hauser, R. The health economics of bladder cancer: a comprehensive review of the published literature. *Pharmacoeconomics.* 2003;21(18):1315-30.

Bustaffa E; Stoccoro A; Bianchi F; Migliore L. Genotoxic and epigenetic mechanisms in arsenic carcinogenicity. *Arch. Toxicol.* 2014 May;88(5):1043-67. doi: 10.1007/s00204-014-1233-7. Epub 2014 Apr 2.

Carreón T; Hein MJ; Hanley KW; Viet SM; Ruder AM. Bladder cancer incidence among workers exposed to o-toluidine, aniline and nitrobenzene at a rubber chemical manufacturing plant. *Occup. Environ. Med.* 2014 Mar;71(3):175-82. doi: 10.1136/oemed-2013-101873.

Catto JW; Abbod MF; Wild PJ; Linkens DA; Pilarsky C; Rehman I; Rosario DJ; Denzinger S; Burger M; Stoehr R; Knuechel R; Hartmann A; Hamdy

FC. The application of artificial intelligence to microarray data: identification of a novel gene signature to identify bladder cancer progression. *Eur. Urol.* 2010 Mar;57(3):398-406. doi: 10.1016/j.eururo.2009.10.029.

Catto JW; Miah S; Owen HC; Bryant H; Myers K; Dudziec E; Larré S; Milo M; Rehman I; Rosario DJ; Di Martino E; Knowles MA; Meuth M; Harris AL; Hamdy FC. Distinct microRNA alterations characterize high- and low-grade bladder cancer. *Cancer Res.* 2009 Nov 1;69(21):8472-81. doi: 10.1158/0008-5472.CAN-09-0744.

Chen G; Wang B; Li H; Ma X; Shi T; Zhang X. Applying narrow-band imaging in complement with white-light imaging cystoscopy in the detection of urothelial carcinoma of the bladder. *Urol Oncol.* 2013 May;31(4):475-9. doi: 10.1016/j.urolonc.2011.02.009.

Chen YT; Chen HW; Domanski D; Smith DS; Liang KH; Wu CC; Chen CL; Chung T; Chen MC; Chang YS; Parker CE; Borchers CH; Yu JS. Multiplexed quantification of 63 proteins in human urine by multiple reaction monitoring-based mass spectrometry for discovery of potential bladder cancer biomarkers. *J. Proteomics.* 2012 Jun 27;75(12):3529-45. doi: 10.1016/j.jprot.2011.12.031.

Chodak GW; Hospelhorn V; Judge SM; Mayforth R; Koeppen H; Sasse J. Increased levels of fibroblast growth factor-like activity in urine from patients with bladder or kidney cancer. *Cancer Res.* 1988 Apr 15;48(8):2083-8.

Chu H; Ma L; Wang M; Shi D; Qin C; Yuan L; Yin C; Zhang Z. The polymorphisms of IL-4, IL-4R and IL-13 genes and bladder cancer risk in a Chinese population: a case-control study. *Mol. Biol. Rep.* 2012 May;39(5):5349-57. doi: 10.1007/s11033-011-1334-9.

Chuang CH; Huang YW; Wu YT. System-level biochip for impedance sensing and programmable manipulation of bladder cancer cells. *Sensors (Basel).* 2011;11(11):11021-35. doi: 10.3390/s111111021.

Chuang CH; Wei CH; Hsu YM; Huang HS; Hsiao FB. Impedance Sensing of Bladder Cancer Cells based on a Single-cell-based DEP Microchip. *IEEE SENSORS 2009 Conference.* 943-947.

Cordeiro ER; Anastasiadis A; Bus MT; Alivizatos G; de la Rosette JJ; de Reijke TM. Is photodynamic diagnosis ready for introduction in urological clinical practice? *Expert Rev. Anticancer Ther.* 2013 Jun;13(6):669-80. doi: 10.1586/era.13.60.

Costa VL; Henrique R; Danielsen SA; Duarte-Pereira S; Eknaes M; Skotheim RI; Rodrigues A; Magalhães JS; Oliveira J; Lothe RA; Teixeira MR;

Jerónimo C; Lind GE. Three epigenetic biomarkers, GDF15, TMEFF2, and VIM, accurately predict bladder cancer from DNA-based analyses of urine samples. *Clin. Cancer Res.* 2010 Dec 1;16(23):5842-51. doi: 10.1158/1078-0432.CCR-10-1312.

de Jong IJ; Pruim J; Elsinga PH; Vaalburg W; Mensink HJ. Visualization of prostate cancer with 11C-choline positron emission tomography. *Eur. Urol.* 2002 Jul;42(1):18-23.

Di Pierro GB; Gulia C; Cristini C; Fraietta G; Marini L; Grande P; Gentile V; Piergentili R. Bladder cancer: a simple model becomes complex. *Curr Genomics.* 2012 Aug;13(5):395-415. doi: 10.2174/138920212801619232.

Ferrís J; Berbel O; Alonso-López J; Garcia J; Ortega JA. Environmental non-occupational risk factors associated with bladder cancer. *Actas Urol Esp.* 2013 Oct;37(9):579-86. doi: 10.1016/j.acuro.2013.02.004.

Frank GA; Zavalishina LE; Andreeva I. Immunohistochemical characteristics and a degree of differentiation of urinary bladder cancer. *Arkh Patol.* 2002;7(6):16–18.

Freedman ND; Silverman DT; Hollenbeck AR; Schatzkin A; Abnet CC. Association between smoking and risk of bladder cancer among men and women. *JAMA.* 2011 Aug 17;306(7):737-45. doi: 10.1001/jama.2011.1142.

Gago-Dominguez M; Castelao JE; Yuan JM; Yu MC; Ross RK. Use of permanent hair dyes and bladder-cancer risk. *Int. J. Cancer.* 2001 Feb 15;91(4):575-9.

Gallagher EJ; LeRoith D. Diabetes, antihyperglycemic medications and cancer risk: smoke or fire? *Curr. Opin. Endocrinol. Diabetes Obes.* 2013 Oct;20(5):485-94. doi: 10.1097/01.med.0000433065.16918.83.

García-Pérez J; Pollán M; Boldo E; Pérez-Gómez B; Aragonés N; Lope V; Ramis R; Vidal E; López-Abente G.Mortality due to lung, laryngeal and bladder cancer in towns lying in the vicinity of combustion installations. *Sci. Total Environ.* 2009 Apr 1;407(8):2593-602. doi: 10.1016/j.scitotenv.2008.12.062.

Gofrit ON; Mishani E; Orevi M; Klein M; Freedman N; Pode D; Shapiro A; Katz R; Libson E; Chisin R. Contribution of 11C-choline positron emission tomography/computerized tomography to preoperative staging of advanced transitional cell carcinoma. *J. Urol.* 2006 Sep;176(3):940-4; discussion 944.

Golka K; Weistenhöfer W. Fire fighters, combustion products, and urothelial cancer. *J. Toxicol. Environ. Health B Crit. Rev.* 2008 Jan;11(1):32-44. doi: 10.1080/10937400701600396.

Gómez-Román JJ; Saenz P; Molina M; Cuevas González J; Escuredo K; Santa Cruz S; Junquera C; Simón L; Martínez A; Gutiérrez Baños JL; López-Brea M; Esparza C; Val-Bernal JF. Fibroblast growth factor receptor 3 is overexpressed in urinary tract carcinomas and modulates the neoplastic cell growth. *Clin Cancer Res*. 2005 Jan 15;11(2 Pt 1):459-65.

Gore JL; Kwan L; Saigal CS; Litwin MS. Marriage and mortality in bladder carcinoma. *Cancer*. 2005 Sep 15;104(6):1188-94.

Grossfeld GD; Carroll PR. Evaluation of asymptomatic microscopic hematuria. *Urol Clin North Am*. 1998 Nov;25(4):661-76.

Gupta S; Bhaijee F; Harmon EP. Mucinous neoplasm arising in a urachal cyst: a first in the pediatric population. *Urology*. 2014 Feb;83(2):455-6. doi: 10.1016/j.urology.2013.09.034.

Hafeez S1; Huddart R. Advances in bladder cancer imaging. *BMC Med*. 2013 Apr 10;11:104. doi: 10.1186/1741-7015-11-104.

Harkirat S; Anand S; Jacob M. Forced diuresis and dual-phase F-fluorodeoxyglucose-PET/CT scan for restaging of urinary bladder cancers. *Indian J Radiol Imaging*. 2010 Feb;20(1):13-9. doi: 10.4103/0971-3026.59746.

Harling M; Schablon A; Schedlbauer G; Dulon M; Nienhaus A. Bladder cancer among hairdressers: a meta-analysis. *Occup. Environ. Med*. 2010 May;67(5):351-8. doi: 10.1136/oem.2009.050195.

Herr HH. Narrow band imaging cystoscopy. *Urol. Oncol*. 2011 Jul-Aug;29(4):353-7.

Holmes E; Wilson ID; Nicholson JK. Metabolic phenotyping in health and disease. *Cell*. 2008 Sep 5;134(5):714-7. doi: 10.1016/j.cell.2008.08.026.

Huang Z; Lin L; Gao Y; Chen Y; Yan X; Xing J; Hang W. Bladder cancer determination via two urinary metabolites: a biomarker pattern approach. *Mol. Cell Proteomics*. 2011 Oct;10(10):M111.007922. doi: 10.1074/mcp. M111.007922.

Jeon M; Kim J; Kim C. Photoacoustic cystography. *J. Vis. Exp*. 2013 Jun 11;(76):e50340. doi: 10.3791/50340.

Kaldor JM1; Day NE; Kittelmann B; Pettersson F; Langmark F; Pedersen D; Prior P; Neal F; Karjalainen S; Bell J; et al. Bladder tumours following chemotherapy and radiotherapy for ovarian cancer: a case-control study. *Int. J. Cancer*. 1995 Sep 27;63(1):1-6.

Kamaya A; Vaithilingam S; Chung BI; Oralkan O; Khuri-Yakub BT. Photoacoustic imaging of the bladder: a pilot study. *J. Ultrasound Med*. 2013 Jul;32(7):1245-50. doi: 10.7863/ultra.32.7.1245.

Ke Z; Lai Y; Ma X; Lil S; Huang W. Diagnosis of bladder cancer from the voided urine specimens using multi-target fluorescence *in situ* hybridization. *Oncol Lett.* 2014 Feb;7(2):325-330.

Keshtkar A; Keshtkar A; Smallwood RH. Electrical impedance spectroscopy and the diagnosis of bladder pathology. *Physiol. Meas.* 2006 Jul;27(7):585-96.

Khalid T; White P; De Lacy Costello B; Persad R; Ewen R; Johnson E; Probert CS; Ratcliffe N. A pilot study combining a GC-sensor device with a statistical model for the identification of bladder cancer from urine headspace. *PLoS One.* 2013 Jul 8;8(7):e69602. doi: 10.1371/ journal. pone.0069602.

Kobayashi S; Koga F; Yoshida S; Masuda H; Ishii C; Tanaka H; Komai Y; Yokoyama M; Saito K; Fujii Y; Kawakami S; Kihara K. Diagnostic performance of diffusion-weighted magnetic resonance imaging in bladder cancer: potential utility of apparent diffusion coefficient values as a biomarker to predict clinical aggressiveness. *Eur Radiol.* 2011 Oct;21(10):2178-86. doi: 10.1007/s00330-011-2174-7. Epub 2011 Jun 18.

Lapini A; Minervini A; Masala A; Schips L; Pycha A; Cindolo L; Giannella R; Martini T; Vittori G; Zani D; Bellomo F; Cosciani Cunico S. A comparison of hexaminolevulinate (Hexvix(®)) fluorescence cystoscopy and white-light cystoscopy for detection of bladder cancer: results of the HeRo observational study. *Surg Endosc.* 2012 Dec;26(12):3634-41. doi: 10.1007/s00464-012-2387-0.

Larsson SC; Orsini N; Wolk A. Milk, milk products and lactose intake and ovarian cancer risk: a meta-analysis of epidemiological studies. *Int. J. Cancer.* 2006 Jan 15;118(2):431-41.

Lee CT; Dunn RL; Williams C; Underwood W 3rd. Racial disparity in bladder cancer: trends in tumor presentation at diagnosis. *J. Urol.* 2006 Sep;176(3):927-33; discussion 933-4.

Lee JW; Lorenzo EI; Ahn B; Oh CK; Kim HJ; Han WK; Kim J; Rha KH. Palpation device for the identification of kidney and bladder cancer: a pilot study. *Yonsei Med. J.* 2011 Sep;52(5):768-72. doi: 10.3349/ ymj.2011.52.5.768.

Lerner SP; Liu H; Wu MF; Thomas YK; Witjes JA. Fluorescence and white light cystoscopy for detection of carcinoma in situ of the urinary bladder. *Urol. Oncol.* 2012 May-Jun;30(3):285-9. doi: 10.1016/ j.urolonc.2010. 09.009.

Letašiová S; Medve'ová A; Šovčíková A; Dušinská M; Volkovová K; Mosoiu C; Bartonová A. Bladder cancer, a review of the environmental risk factors. *Environ Health*. 2012 Jun 28;11 Suppl 1:S11. doi: 10.1186/1476-069X-11-S1-S11.

Li QY; Tang J; He EH; Li YM; Zhou Y; Zhang X; Chen G. Clinical utility oft hree-dimensional contrast-enhanced ultrasound in the differentiation between noninvasive and invasive neoplasms of urinary bladder. *Eur. J. Radiol.* 2012. 81:2936–2942.

Liu IJ; Lai YH; Espiritu JI; Segall GM; Srinivas S; Nino-Murcia M; Terris MK. Evaluation of fluorodeoxyglucose positron emission tomography imaging in metastatic transitional cell carcinoma with and without prior chemotherapy. *Urol. Int*. 2006;77(1):69-75.

Lotan Y; Daudon M; Bruyère F; Talaska G; Strippoli G; Johnson RJ; Tack I. Impact of fluid intake in the prevention of urinary system diseases: a brief review. *Curr. Opin. Nephrol. Hypertens*. 2013 May;22 Suppl 1:S1-10. doi: 10.1097/MNH.0b013e328360a268.

MacVicar AD. Bladder cancer staging. *BJU Int*. 2000 Jul;86 Suppl 1:111-22.

Mao Q; Lin Y; Zheng X; Qin J; Yang K; Xie L. A meta-analysis of alcohol intake and risk of bladder cancer. *Cancer Causes Control*. 2010 Nov;21(11):1843-50. doi: 10.1007/s10552-010-9611-9.

Mao QQ; Dai Y; Lin YW; Qin J; Xie LP; Zheng XY. Milk consumption and bladder cancer risk: a meta-analysis of published epidemiological studies. *Nutr Cancer*. 2011 Nov;63(8):1263-71. doi: 10.1080/01635581.2011.614716.

Mariotto AB; Yabroff KR; Shao Y; Feuer EJ; Brown ML. Projections of the Cost of Cancer Care in the United States: 2010–2020. *J Natl Cancer Inst*. 2011 Jan 19;103(2):117-28. doi: 10.1093/jnci/djq495.

Martingano P; Stacul F; Cavallaro M; Casagrande F; Cernic S; Belgrano M; Cova M. 64-Slice CT urography: 30 months of clinical experience. *Radiol Med*. 2010 Sep;115(6):920-35. doi: 10.1007/s11547-010-0567-3.

May M; Bastian PJ; Brookman-May S; Fritsche HM; Tilki D; Otto W; Bolenz C; Gilfrich C; Trojan L; Herrmann E; Moritz R; Tiemann A; Müller SC; Ellinger J; Buchner A; Stief CG; Wieland WF; Höfner T; Hohenfellner M; Haferkamp A; Roigas J; Zacharias M; Nuhn P; Burger M. Gender-specific differences in cancer-specific survival after radical cystectomy for patients with urothelial carcinoma of the urinary bladder in pathologic tumor stage T4a. *Urol. Oncol.* 2013 Oct; 31(7):1141-7. doi: 10.1016/ j.urolonc.2011.09.011.

Mazdak H; Yazdekhasti F; Movahedian A; Mirkheshti N; Shafieian M. The comparative study of serum iron, copper, and zinc levels between bladder cancer patients and a control group. *Int Urol Nephrol.* 2010 Mar;42(1):89-93. doi: 10.1007/s11255-009-9583-4.

Mhawech-Fauceglia P; Fischer G; Alvarez V Jr; Ahmed A; Herrmann FR. Predicting outcome in minimally invasive (T1a and T1b) urothelial bladder carcinoma using a panel of biomarkers: a high throughput tissue microarray analysis. *BJU Int.* 2007 Nov;100(5):1182-7.

Mlcochova H; Hezova R; Stanik M; Slaby O. Urine microRNAs as potential noninvasive biomarkers in urologic cancers. *Urol Oncol.* 2014 Jan;32(1):41.e1-9. doi: 10.1016/j.urolonc.2013.04.011.

Moonen PM; Merkx GF; Peelen P; Karthaus HF; Smeets DF; Witjes JA. UroVysion compared with cytology and quantitative cytology in the surveillance of non-muscle-invasive bladder cancer. *Eur. Urol.* 2007 May;51(5):1275-80; discussion 1280.

Mostafa MH; Sheweita SA; O'Connor PJ. Relationship between schistosomiasis and bladder cancer. *Clin. Microbiol. Rev.* 1999 Jan;12(1):97-111.

Murta-Nascimento C; Schmitz-Dräger BJ; Zeegers MP; Steineck G; Kogevinas M; Real FX; Malats N. Epidemiology of urinary bladder cancer: from tumor development to patient's death.*World J. Urol.* 2007 Jun;25(3):285-95.

Nieder AM; Porter MP; Soloway MS. Radiation therapy for prostate cancer increases subsequent risk of bladder and rectal cancer: a population based cohort study. *J. Urol.* 2008 Nov;180(5):2005-9; discussion 2009-10. doi: 10.1016/j.juro.2008.07.038.

Oberoi S; Barchowsky A; Wu F. The global burden of disease for skin, lung and bladder cancer caused by arsenic in food. *Cancer Epidemiol. Biomarkers Prev.* 2014 May 3. [Epub ahead of print]

Ogaya Pinies G; Herranz Amo F; Escribano Patiño G; Lledó García E; Molina Escudero R; Husillos Alonso A; Hernandez Fernandez C. Urachal adenocarcinoma. Case report and bibliographic review. *Arch. Esp. Urol.* 2012 May;65(4):498-501.

Osman I; Bajorin DF; Sun TT; Zhong H; Douglas D; Scattergood J; Zheng R; Han M; Marshall KW; Liew CC. Novel blood biomarkers of human urinary bladder cancer. *Clin. Cancer Res.* 2006 Jun 1;12(11 Pt 1):3374-80.

Oude Elferink P; Witjes JA. Blue-light cystoscopy in the evaluation of non-muscle-invasive bladder cancer. *Ther Adv. Urol.* 2014 Feb;6(1):25-33.

Padhani AR; Husband JE. Dynamic contrast-enhanced MRI studies in oncology with an emphasis on quantification, validation and human studies. *Clin Radiol.* 2001 Aug;56(8):607-20.

Pelucchi C; Bosetti C; Negri E; Malvezzi M; La Vecchia C. Mechanisms of disease: The epidemiology of bladder cancer. *Nat. Clin. Pract. Urol.* 2006 Jun;3(6):327-40.

Pelucchi C; Galeone C; Tramacere I; Bagnardi V; Negri E; Islami F; Scotti L; Bellocco R; Corrao G; Boffetta P; La Vecchia C. Alcohol drinking and bladder cancer risk: a meta-analysis. *Ann. Oncol.* 2012 Jun;23(6):1586-93. doi: 10.1093/annonc/mdr460.

Peumery JJ. Histoire illustrée du diabète: de l'antiquité à nos jours, Parigi, Editions Roger Dacosta, 1987. ISBN 10: 2851280694 / ISBN 13: 9782851280695.

Pichler BJ; Kolb A; Nägele T; Schlemmer HP. PET/MRI: paving the way for the next generation of clinical multimodality imaging applications. *J Nucl Med.* 2010 Mar;51(3):333-6. doi: 10.2967/jnumed.109.061853.

Piergentili R; Carradori S; Gulia C; De Monte C; Cristini C; Grande P; Santini E; Gentile V; Di Pierro GB. Bladder cancer: innovative approaches beyond the diagnosis. *Curr. Med. Chem.* 2014;21(20):2219-36.

Qin LQ; Xu JY; Wang PY; Tong J; Hoshi K. Milk consumption is a risk factor for prostate cancer in Western countries: evidence from cohort studies. *Asia Pac. J. Clin. Nutr.* 2007 16(3):467-76.

Reinert T; Modin C; Castano FM; Lamy P; Wojdacz TK; Hansen LL; Wiuf C; Borre M; Dyrskjøt L; Orntoft TF. Comprehensive genome methylation analysis in bladder cancer: identification and validation of novel methylated genes and application of these as urinary tumor markers. *Clin Cancer Res.* 2011 Sep 1;17(17):5582-92. doi: 10.1158/1078-0432.CCR-10-2659.

Ren H; Park KC; Pan R; Waltzer WC; Shroyer KR; Pan Y. Early detection of carcinoma in situ of the bladder: a comparative study of white light cystoscopy, narrow band imaging, 5-ALA fluorescence cystoscopy and 3-dimensional optical coherence tomography. *J. Urol.* 2012 Mar;187(3):1063-70. doi: 10.1016/j.juro.2011.10.131.

Ro JY; Staerkel GA; Ayala AG. Cytologic and histologic features of superficial bladder cancer. *Urol Clin. North Am.* 1992 Aug;19(3):435-53.

Ros MM; Gago-Dominguez M; Aben KK; Bueno-de-Mesquita HB; Kampman E; Vermeulen SH; Kiemeney LA. Personal hair dye use and the risk of bladder cancer: a case-control study from The Netherlands. *Cancer Causes Control.* 2012 Jul;23(7):1139-48. doi: 10.1007/s10552-012-9982-1.

Roy S; Parwani AV. Adenocarcinoma of the urinary bladder. *Arch Pathol Lab Med.* 2011 Dec;135(12):1601-5. doi: 10.5858/arpa.2009-0713-RS.

Saksena MA; Dahl DM; Harisinghani MG. New imaging modalities in bladder cancer. *World J. Urol.* 2006 Nov;24(5):473-80.

Schiffer E; Vlahou A; Petrolekas A; Stravodimos K; Tauber R; Geschwend JE; Neuhaus J; Stolzenburg JU; Conaway MR; Mischak H; Theodorescu D. Prediction of muscle-invasive bladder cancer using urinary proteomics. *Clin Cancer Res.* 2009 Aug 1;15(15):4935-43. doi: 10.1158/1078-0432.CCR-09-0226. Epub 2009 Jul 14.

Scosyrev E; Trivedi D; Messing E. Female bladder cancer: incidence, treatment, and outcome. *Curr. Opin. Urol.* 2010 Sep;20(5):404-8. doi: 10.1097/MOU.0b013e32833c7a9b.

Shariat SF; Sfakianos JP; Droller MJ; Karakiewicz PI; Meryn S; Bochner BH. The effect of age and gender on bladder cancer: a critical review of the literature. *BJU Int.* 2010 Feb;105(3):300-8. doi: 10.1111/j.1464-410X.2009.09076.x.

Shariat SF; Youssef RF; Gupta A; Chade DC; Karakiewicz PI; Isbarn H; Jeldres C; Sagalowsky AI; Ashfaq R; Lotan Y. Association of angiogenesis related markers with bladder cancer outcomes and other molecular markers. *J. Urol.* 2010 May;183(5):1744-50. doi: 10.1016/j.juro.2010.01.018.

Shen C; Wu J; Hsu C; Jou Y; Lin C; Wang M; Wu S; Chan M; Chiang M; Fang C; Chang D. The high incidence of JC virus infection in urothelial carcinoma tissue in Taiwan. *J. Med. Virol.* 2011;7(12):2191–2199. doi: 10.1002/jmv.22240.

Shen Y; Liu Y; Liu S; Zhang A. The association between -330T/G polymorphism of interleukin 2 gene and bladder cancer. *DNA Cell Biol.* 2012 Jun;31(6):983-7. doi: 10.1089/dna.2011.1476.

Shi Z; Wei Q; Zhang M; She J. MicroRNAs in bladder cancer: expression profiles, biological functions, regulation, and clinical implications. *Crit Rev Eukaryot Gene Expr.* 2014;24(1):55-75.

Sievert, KD; Amend, B; Nagele, U; Schilling, D; Bedke, J; Horstmann, M; Hennenlotter, J; Kruck, S; Stenzl, A. Economic aspects of bladder cancer: what are the benefits and costs? *World J. Urol.* 2009 Jun;27(3):295-300. doi: 10.1007/s00345-009-0395-z.

Spratlin JL; Serkova NJ; Eckhardt SG. Clinical applications of metabolomics in oncology: a review. *Clin. Cancer Res.* 2009 Jan 15;15(2):431-40. doi: 10.1158/1078-0432.CCR-08-1059.

Svatek, RS; Hollenbeck BK; Holmäng S; Lee R; Kim SP; Stenzl A; Lotan Y. The Economics of Bladder Cancer: Costs and Considerations of Caring for This Disease. *Eur. Urol.* 2014 Jan 21. pii: S0302-2838(14)00018-9. doi: 10.1016/j.eururo.2014.01.006.

Takeuchi M; Sasaki S; Ito M; Okada S; Takahashi S; Kawai T; Suzuki K; Oshima H; Hara M; Shibamoto Y. Urinary bladder cancer: diffusion-weighted MR imaging--accuracy for diagnosing T stage and estimating histologic grade. *Radiology*. 2009 Apr; 251(1):112-21. doi: 10.1148 /radiol.2511080873.

Taylor NJ; Baddeley H; Goodchild KA; Powell ME; Thoumine M; Culver LA; Stirling JJ; Saunders MI; Hoskin PJ; Phillips H; Padhani AR; Griffiths JR. BOLD MRI of human tumor oxygenation during carbogen breathing. *J. Magn Reson Imaging*. 2001 Aug;14(2):156-63.

Thoeny HC; Triantafyllou M; Birkhaeuser FD; Froehlich JM; Tshering DW; Binser T; Fleischmann A; Vermathen P; Studer UE. Combined ultrasmall superparamagnetic particles of iron oxide-enhanced and diffusion-weighted magnetic resonance imaging reliably detect pelvic lymph node metastases in normal-sized nodes of bladder and prostate cancer patients. *Eur. Urol.* 2009 Apr;55(4):761-9. doi: 10.1016/j.eururo.2008.12.034.

Thomsen HS. Nephrogenic systemic fibrosis: history and epidemiology. *Radiol. Clin. North Am.* 2009 Sep;47(5):827-31, vi. doi: 10.1016/ j.rcl.2009.05.003.

Tölle A; Jung M; Rabenhorst S; Kilic E; Jung K; Weikert S. Identification of microRNAs in blood and urine as tumour markers for the detection of urinary bladder cancer. *Oncol. Rep.* 2013 Oct;30(4):1949-56. doi: 10.3892/or.2013.2621.

Travis LB; Curtis RE; Glimelius B; Holowaty EJ; Van Leeuwen FE; Lynch CF; Hagenbeek A; Stovall M; Banks PM; Adami J; et al. Bladder and kidney cancer following cyclophosphamide therapy for non-Hodgkin's lymphoma. *J. Natl. Cancer Inst.* 1995 Apr 5;87(7):524-30.

Tritschler S; Mosler C; Tilki D; Buchner A; Stief C; Graser A. Interobserver variability limits exact preoperative staging by computed tomography in bladder cancer. *Urology*. 2012 Jun;79(6):1317-21. doi: 10.1016/j. urology.2012.01.040.

Tseng CH. A review on thiazolidinediones and bladder cancer in human studies. *J. Environ. Sci. Health C Environ. Carcinog Ecotoxicol. Rev*. 2014;32(1):1-45. doi: 10.1080/10590501.2014.877645.

Tuncbilek N; Kaplan M; Altaner S; Atakan IH; Süt N; Inci O; Demir MK. Value of dynamic contrast-enhanced MRI and correlation with tumor angiogenesis in bladder cancer. *AJR Am. J. Roentgenol.* 2009 Apr;192(4):949-55. doi: 10.2214/AJR.08.1332.

Underwood W 3rd; Dunn RL; Williams C; Lee CT. Gender and geographic influence on the racial disparity in bladder cancer mortality in the US. *J. Am. Coll. Surg.* 2006 Feb;202(2):284-90.

van Kessel KE; Kompier LC; de Bekker-Grob EW; Zuiverloon TC; Vergouwe Y; Zwarthoff EC; Steyerberg EW. FGFR3 mutation analysis in voided urine samples to decrease cystoscopies and cost in nonmuscle invasive bladder cancer surveillance: a comparison of 3 strategies. *J. Urol.* 2013 May;189(5):1676-81. doi: 10.1016/j.juro.2012.11.005.

Veerla S; Lindgren D; Kvist A; Frigyesi A; Staaf J; Persson H; Liedberg F; Chebil G; Gudjonsson S; Borg A; Månsson W; Rovira C; Höglund M. MiRNA expression in urothelial carcinomas: important roles of miR-10a, miR-222, miR-125b, miR-7 and miR-452 for tumor stage and metastasis, and frequent homozygous losses of miR-31. *Int. J. Cancer.* 2009 May 1;124(9):2236-42. doi: 10.1002/ijc.24183.

West H. Pee a Rainbow: Scientist Snaps Shot of Colorful Urine. Interview by Becky Oskin published by *LifeScience online Magazine*, June 22, 2013. Accessed May 2014. http://www.livescience.com/37664-human-urine-colors-rainbow.html

Willis CM; Church SM; Guest CM; Cook WA; McCarthy N; Bransbury AJ; Church MR; Church JC. Olfactory detection of human bladder cancer by dogs: proof of principle study. *BMJ.* 2004 Sep 25;329(7468):712.

Xie Z; Roberts W; Carson P; Liu X; Tao C; Wang X. Evaluation of bladder microvasculature with high-resolution photoacoustic imaging. *Opt. Lett.* 2011 Dec 15;36(24):4815-7. doi: 10.1364/OL.36.004815.

Yang M. A current global view of environmental and occupational cancers. *J. Environ. Sci. Health C Environ. Carcinog Ecotoxicol Rev.* 2011 Jul;29(3):223-49. doi: 10.1080/10590501.2011.601848.

Yee DS; Ishill NM; Lowrance WT; Herr HW; Elkin EB. Ethnic differences in bladder cancer survival. *Urology.* 2011 Sep;78(3):544-9. doi: 10.1016/j.urology.2011.02.042.

Zackrisson S; van de Ven SM; Gambhir SS. Light in and sound out: emerging translational strategies for photoacoustic imaging. *Cancer Res.* 2014 Feb 15;74(4):979-1004. doi: 10.1158/0008-5472.CAN-13-2387. Epub 2014 Feb 10.

Zuiverloon TC; Beukers W; van der Keur KA; Munoz JR; Bangma CH; Lingsma HF; Eijkemans MJ; Schouten JP; Zwarthoff EC. A methylation assay for the detection of non-muscle-invasive bladder cancer (NMIBC) recurrences in voided urine. *BJU Int.* 2012 Mar;109(6):941-8. doi: 10.1111/j.1464-410X.2011.10428.x.

In: Bladder Cancer
Editor: Samantha Haggerty
ISBN: 978-1-63321-666-2

Chapter 3

BLADDER CANCER IN PEDIATRIC PATIENTS

Santiago Vallasciani*[1], *Giacinto Marrocco*[2], *Caterina Gulia*[3], *Andrea Zangari*[2] *and Roberto Piergentili*[4]

[1]UOSD di Urologia Pediatrica, Policlinico Maggiore, Milano, Italia
[2]UOC di Chirurgia ed Urologia Pediatrica, Azienda Ospedaliera San Camillo-Forlanini, Roma, Italia
[3]Dipartimento di Scienze Ginecologico-Ostetriche e Scienze Urologiche, Policlinico Umberto I, Sapienza - Università di Roma, Italia
[4]Istituto di Biologia, Medicina Molecolare e Nanobiotecnologie del CNR; Dipartimento di Biologia e Biotecnologie, Sapienza - Università di Roma, Italia

ABSTRACT

Lower urinary tract malignancies are very rare in pediatric age and highly uncommon in the first two decades of life; indeed, according to most available reports, their incidence among all affected patients if far lower that 1%. In fact, the sum of all patients for all bladder tumours in available scientific literature is just a few hundreds. These pathologies resemble in some instances their adult counterparts, such as painless macroscopic haematuria as first symptom, the males are more affected than females, the familiarity, the relationship with specific chemicals

* Corresponding Author: RP – roberto.piergentili@uniroma1.it.

such as those linked to pollution. Nonetheless, there are other aspects of bladder cancers (BC) in children that show specific characteristics: (i) pediatric BC are usually unifocal; (ii) despite delayed diagnosis due to the unexpected pathology, consequently driving towards a different initial diagnosis, children usually show lower grade and stage cancers at presentation, compared to adults; (iii) their prognosis is, in general, relatively good compared to that of elder people; (iv) the recurrence rate is very low; (v) the tumors usually show an indolent behavior; (vi) although males are more affected, the male-to-female ratio shows an age-dependent value, with males being more affected at younger ages. Taken together, these facts suggest that BC in young patients is different from that of elderly people. Moreover, also its treatment needs a different approach, since in children and adolescents it is very important to preserve fertility and sexual performances. In this report, similarities and differences in BC between young and adults will be discussed, and alternative therapeutic approaches will be illustrated.

INTRODUCTION

It is generally accepted that bladder cancer (BC) is an age-related disease. Indeed, the USA National Cancer Institute (NCI) website (accession: May 2014) (http://www.cancer.gov) reports that more than 70% of affected patients are at least 65 years old, and the peak of the incidence falls in the age frame 75-84 (>30% of total new cases), with a median age at diagnosis of 73 years.

Table 1. Age-Specific SEER 18 Areas Incidence Rates, years 2007-2011, according to SEER web site, all races (direct link in text body). Rates are per 100,000 and are age-adjusted to the 2000 US Standard Population (19 age groups - Census P25-1130). Dash: statistic not shown; rate based on less than 16 cases for the time interval

Age at Diagnosis	Both Sexes	Males	Females
<1	-	-	-
1-4	-	-	-
5-9	-	-	-
10-14	-	-	-
15-19	0.1	-	-
20-24	0.2	0.3	-
25-29	0.4	0.6	0.2
30-34	0.7	1.1	0.4

The United States SEER (Surveillance, Epidemiology, and End Results) Program reports that patients aged ≤20 years represent the 0.1% of all BC new cases (SEER 18 2007-2011, All Races, Both Sexes) and extremely rare fatal episodes. These numbers raise to 0.4% when considering the age interval 20-34 years for new cases, and 0.1% for mortality (percentage among all diagnosed cases). The analysis of more discrete age intervals are reported in Table 1, as illustrated in SEER web site (http://seer.cancer.gov/csr/1975_2011/browse_csr.php?sectionSEL=27&pageSEL=sect_27_table.07.html). As shown, BC diagnosed below the age of 14 can be considered sporadic.

RHABDOMYOSARCOMA (RMS)

This neoplasm is relatively rare in absolute terms, accounting for 4–8% of the malignant tumors in patients younger than 15 years of age (Chigurupati et al., 2002; Merguerian et al., 2007). It is not specific for the localization - it may develop in several body districts such as head, neck, abdomen, extremities. Nonetheless, the genitourinary tract is its second most usual site of localization in children, and accounting for up to 20% of all cases (Heinzelmann et al., 2011). RMS is the most frequent pediatric genitourinary tumor, showing an incidence of 4.5 cases per million children/adolescents per year (Ognjanovic et al., 2009). Of them, it is estimated that approximately 20% of primary RMS form in the urinary bladder (Lott et al., 2007). Thus, overall, RMS is the most common tumor of the bladder in children (Leuschner et al., 2001). Nearly 75% of genitourinary RMS cases are diagnosed before the age of 5 years, with a male to female ratio of 3.3:1 (Merguerian et al., 2007). Symptoms include urinary tract obstruction, hematuria, and abdominal mass; usually, at presentation it is already larger than 5 cm and with invasive properties. A neonatal alveolar subtype has been described in literature, having multiple cutaneous metastases and poor prognosis (Merguerian et al., 2007), making it the most common pediatric neoplasm able to metastasize to the skin (Wesche et al., 2000). Rhabdomyosarcoma presents two peaks of incidence: the first, which accounts for more than 50% of cases, during the first decade of life, especially in the age range 2-4 years; the second during adolescence, mostly in 15-19 years old adolescents. With the exception cited above about the neonatal subtype, these two peaks also roughly correspond to different histopathologic variants of the sarcoma itself. The former is mainly embryonal and can be classified into two subtypes, namely spindle cell and botryoid.

Spindle cell sarcoma is common in paratesticular lesions, whereas botryoid lesions are polypoid masses that fill the lumen of bladder and vagina (Dasgupta and Rodeberg, 2012). The alveolar sarcoma is instead more frequent in the second age range (Qualman et al., 1998). Embryonal RMS rarely metastasizes and responds well to current therapy; instead, the alveolar hystotype is more aggressive and with poorer prognosis both in adolescents and adults (Newton et al., 1995).

This neoplasm may be part of the phenotypic spectrum of several syndromes, including neurofibromatosis, Costello syndrome, Gorlin's basal cell nevus syndrome, Rubinstein-Taybi syndrome, Down syndrome, Beckwith-Wiedemann syndrome (BWS), fetal alcohol syndrome, and Li-Fraumeni syndrome (Merguerian et al., 2007). The Li-Fraumeni syndrome is usually associated to a dominant TP53 mutation; notably, changes in this gene are very frequent in BC bioptic samples also in BC affected adults (Di Pierro et al., 2012). RMS derives from the embryonic mesenchymal cells generating the striated musculature; since it resembles evidence of skeletal muscle differentiation and may occur in sites where skeletal muscle is not found, it likely develops from aberrant myogenic differentiation. Consequently, several genes involved in this process are either deregulated or mutated in RMS specimens (Merguerian et al., 2007). To date, genes related to RMS formation encompass *MyoD* and *myogenin* (transcription factors involved in muscle differentiation), *MDM2* (encoding a TP53 inhibitor), *PAX3* and *PAX7* (transcription factors involved in the development of mesenchymal precursors), *EWS* (Ewing's sarcoma gene), *H19* (an RNA molecule widely expressed during fetal development), *CDKN1C* (a cyclin-dependent kinase inhibitor that negatively regulates cell cycle progression, expressed also in the skeletal muscle), *STIM1/GOK* (a calcium sensor), various *RAS* gene family members (signal transducers) (Merguerian et al., 2007) and *SMARCB1/INI1/BAF47* (a chromatin structure regulator) (Savage et al., 2012).

Diagnosis is usually achieved by pelvic and renal ultrasonography, allowing the recognition of an abdominal mass which may be either hyper- or hypo-echoic. The extension of the disease and the identification of possible metastatic foci are normally performed by nuclear magnetic resonance (NMR) or computer-aided tomography (CT) imaging. Metastases may target several organs, including primarily lymph nodes, lungs, bone and, subsequently, bone marrow and liver (Kim et al., 2000). In particular, bone metastases are visualized as lytic lesions (Kim et al., 2000); bone marrow involvement at diagnosis is indicative of poor prognosis, with less than 10% survival (Merguerian et al., 2007). Tumor confirmation derives from direct histologic analysis of specimens, with the samples obtained either by cystoscopy or by needle biopsy. Nuclear image morphometry has been used as well for diagnosis and resulted quite affordable for differential diagnosis with other neoplasms, with the exception of retinoblastoma on FNA (Brahmi et al., 2001).

In the last decades, the outcome of children affected by this tumor has greatly improved, and overall 10-year survival is around 80% for all genitourinary RMS, and 66% for bladder/prostate sites (Punyko et al., 2005). Pediatric patients need an integrated approach, requiring surgery, chemotherapy and radiotherapy, particularly because of RMS high sensitivity to chemotherapeutic agents. However, due to connected complications and morbidity, the optimal time, extent and intensity of these treatments for children remain controversial (Walterhouse and Watson, 2007; Wu et al., 2009). Cystectomy, if practicable, is generally recommended (Filipas et al., 2004), yet surgery applied to children may present several challenges, considering both the physical body dimensions, and the need to preserve as much as possible physiological functions in the very long term; consequently, radical cystectomy should be avoided, unless tumor localization discourages partial bladder removal. Instead, other Authors prefer chemotherapy as a first line intervention, by suggesting vincristine, dactinomycin and cyclophosphamide (or ifosfamide as an alternative for the last one) (Heinzelmann et al., 2011). It must be remembered, however, that the toxicity of such molecules is high, especially in children. As a matter of fact, among side effects, several manuscripts report renal toxicity (particularly in very young patients), myelosuppression, infections, hematuria, delayed pubertal development, growth retardation, secondary malignancies and recurrences/relapses (Merguerian et al., 2007). As expected, children with both high stage neoplasm and large primary lesion at diagnosis (>5 cm) show the highest risk for late events. In this therapeutic context, the use of radiations is mostly aimed at residual tumor treatment, after either front-line surgery or chemotherapy (Punyko et al., 2005; Walterhouse and Watson, 2007). However, according to the results of several studies, also this approach should be used considering patients' age, tumor site, and amount of residual tumor. Standard available protocols suggest a dose of 40 Gy for microscopic residues (with a treatment margin of 2 cm) and 45-55 Gy if the tumor shows adverse characteristics, such as large size, unfavorable site or lymph nodes involvement (Merguerian et al., 2007). Recently, a group from Ankara treated two RMS patients using transurethral resection (TUR) - although this technique is not an established method in this context - followed by chemotherapy (Ozturk et al., 2013). In this case, they used TUR to remove gross tumor tissue, and chemotherapy (VAC protocol for 43 weeks) to treat microscopic residual lesions; the follow-up of 51 and 49 months for the two patients, respectively, allowed excluding any recurrence, indicating that this alternative approach may be useful at least in some selected cases.

Transitional Cell Papilloma (TCP) and Carcinoma (TCC)

TCP are benign bladder tumors of epithelial origin (Gites, 1979). It is very rare and, upon histological analysis, it is composed of a normal exophytic urothelium organized on a tender stalk of fibrovascular nature (Epstein et al., 1998). However, its classification is not straightforward among specialists. Indeed, some consider it a papilloma *tout-court*, while others classify it as a "papillary urothelial neoplasm of low malignant potential (PUNLMP)" (Thomas et al., 2006), which anyhow makes little difference in terms of management. For some Authors, TCP is instead a precocious phase of TCC development (TCC of grade 0 or 1) (Melicow, 1955). In children, this neoplasm is rare, but its rate of recurrence is relatively high - a review of the literature (Thomas et al., 2006) reports 14 children affected (including the case described in the cited manuscript), 6 of which (>40%) with at least one recurrence. Thus, despite its benign nature, children must be followed carefully, since highly recurrent forms may be fatal because of organ function impairment (Chandy et al., 1975). The cause of such an high rate of recurrence is currently unknown, but it is unlikely that it may be simply ascribed to incomplete removal, owing to the relative high number of unrelated cases. In most patients (8/14) it formed next to one ureteric orifice; some Authors consequently related its development to local, long-term inflammations (Thomas et al., 2006). Diagnosis in all cases may be successfully performed by ultrasound imaging, and its removal is normally performed using an endoscopic approach and fulguration (Thomas et al., 2006).

TCC is generally considered exceptional under age 10, and in any case rare among 10 to 20 years old patients. The few available data indicate that its incidence is around 0.4% among all epithelial BC in patients of this age range (Jayadpour and Mostofi, 1969). Recent reviews of the entire available literature (Lerena et al., 2010; Dénes et al., 2013) report a total of ca. 150 patients aged at most 20 years; of them, only about 20% aged less than 10. The males to females sex ratio among TCC patients is 3:1, and whites seem more prone than blacks to the disease (39 times higher incidence) (Madgar et al., 1988). Although several risk factors had been reported in literature for adults, either genetic or non genetic (smoking, occupational exposure to aniline dyes) (Di Pierro et al., 2012), to date none of these had been clearly recognized in pediatric literature (Giedl et al., 2006; Lerena et al., 2010; Paner et al., 2011). TCC pediatric patients are usually (80%) diagnosed after episodes of - sometimes intermittent - macroscopic haematuria, yet other symptoms may be present such as urinary tract infections and/or irritations (15%) and microscopic hematuria (8%); dysuria is atypical in these children (Hoenig et al., 1996).

Diagnosis in these situations may be delayed because of the unexpected disease and generally underestimated symptoms (Ruiz et al., 2009). First-line imaging usually involves ultrasonography (Lerena et al., 2010), while intravenous pyelography and computer-aided tomography may fail to identify small tumors. Definitive assessment of the disease relies mainly on cystoscopy, since cytology is not sufficiently established in this age range because of TCC low grade (Hoenig et al., 1996; Ruiz et al., 2009). Despite these diagnostic problems, patients have good chances of a positive outcome, since in 75% of TCC cases, invasiveness is either minimal or completely absent (grade I or papillomas), and only 3% show invasiveness through *lamina propria*; moreover, in more than 90% of cases, TCC are represented by single lesions (Merguerian et al., 2007). In these patients surgery is the standard removal approach, through endoscopic resection of all localized lesions. Follow-up is normally performed by ultrasonography, and recurrences are found in about 13% of patients; secondary invasiveness involving muscular tissues affects 10-15% of patients (Bujons et al., 2013).

LEIOMYOMA AND LEIOMYOSARCOMA

Leiomyomas are benign, non-infiltrative, smooth-muscle tumors that usually form in the uterine and bladder walls. Their histology is quite typical: they are diffusely immunoreactive for smooth muscle actin, muscle-specific actin, desmin, and vimentin; instead, they are normally negative for both cytokeratin and S100 protein (Chen et al., 2012). These tumors are relatively common in adults, and are often found incidentally during surgery aimed at other targets. Mesenchymal tumors of the urinary bladder are heterogeneous and constitute 1%-5% of all bladder neoplasms (Matsushima et al., 2010). Of them, leiomyoma is the most common type, totaling 0.43% of all cases (Blasco-Casares et al., 1995); in adults, it mainly involves women (75%, mean age 44 years) (Goluboff et al., 1994). Pediatric bladder leyomiomas are instead extremely rare: in literature, only two cases are reported, one involving an 11 years old girl (Mutchler and Gorder, 1972) and the second found in a 6 years old boy (Chen et al., 2012); both were treated by open surgery. The male patient underwent ultrasonography and tomography, but the lesion could not be clearly distinguished from several other diseases, and open surgery plus histopathologic examination was necessary for ultimate diagnosis and to rule out the presence of a leiomyosarcoma. Because of the lack of data, pathophysiology of pediatric leiomyoma is currently unknown, and only theories are available in literature about its formation in adults (Cornella et al., 1997; Teran and Gambrell, 1989; Furuhashi and Suganuma, 2002).

Leiomyosarcoma is considered the malignant counterpart of leiomyoma, although the former does not derive from the latter. They account for only 0.1% of all bladder cancers (Perdersen-Bjergaard et al., 1995). There is no general agreement in literature about the histopathologic differences between bladder leiomyoma and leiomyosarcoma. Leiomyomas are usually well-differentiated, while leiomyosarcomas may be either well- or poorly-differentiated, the former resembling leiomyomas to a certain extent. Poorly differentiated leiomyosarcomas show extensive atypia and pleomorphism. Martin and co-workers (2002) suggest that leiomyoma is the non-infiltrative, smooth muscle tumor lacking mitotic activity, cytologic atypia, and necrosis. In adults, leiomyosarcomas are rarer than leiomyomas. These sarcomas have a tendency to metastasize early, often to the lung, and to recur after surgery. In pediatric patients, these neoplasms are even rarer, accounting for less than 2% of all soft tissue sarcomas; as their adult counterparts, they are usually removed by surgery. Leiomyosarcoma may arise as a secondary tumor in patients treated for retinoblastoma (Brucker et al., 2006), but in these cases the rarity of this lesion and the lack of a uniform staging system has made their treatment empiric (Parekh et al., 2002). A subtype of this neoplasm is the urachal leiomyosarcoma, of which to date only 8 cases had been reported, mainly in children and young adults (Noyes and Vinson, 1981). The last case reported in literature occurred in a 12 years old boy (Kim et al., 2007). Also for this subtype, indications about diagnosis and treatment are problematic due to the paucity of available data.

Urachal Adenocarcinoma (UA)

Urachal anomalies are relatively rare in clinical practice because of their usually asymptomatic nature. Estimations on their true prevalence based on 122 corpses autopsy revealed tubular urachal remnants in 32% of the adult bladders (Schubert et al., 1982). Urachal tumors are generally divided into benign adenomas and malignant adenocarcinomas. The UA usually forms in the juxtavesical segment of the urachus, then progresses towards the bladder; it is typically mucin-producing or colloid. This neoplasm is one of the rarest bladder tumors, accounting for 0.17%-0.34% of all vesical lesions (Merguerian et al., 2007). Despite this, several reports are present in literature describing pediatric cases (Merguerian et al., 2007; Gupta et al., 2014). Indeed, adenocarcinomas of urachal origin account for 20%-30% of all bladder adenocarcinomas, which in turn are almost 5% of all bladder tumors (Siefker-Radtke, 2012). First-line intervention is usually surgery, yet the prognosis is unfavorable because delayed detection and diagnosis may allow the cancer to easily spread, thanks to its peculiar localization (Merguerian et al., 2007).

Adenocarcinoma of the Exstrophied Bladder

Classic bladder exstrophy is a rare congenital malformation occurring with an incidence of about 1 in 50 000 live births and an even male to female ratio (Nelson et al., 2005). Young patients affected by exstrophied bladder have higher risks of developing a BC. Indeed, BC incidence for them is much higher than that of the normal population under 40 years old (Smeulders and Woodhouse 2001). Most reported cases occurred in patients with defunctioned bladders via urinary diversion during childhood, and the risk of malignancy is lower in patients with a functioning reconstructed bladder (Paulhac et al., 1999). Histologically, this cancer shows colonic epithelium replacing normal bladder tissue, and producing colon-specific mucin and carcinoembryonic antigen; moreover, the colonic epithelium frequently shows dysplasia and areas of colonic exophytic adenocarcinoma (Merguerian et al., 2007). Exstrophied bladder also shows typical polypoid lesions having deep penetrating nests of urothelium or cysts and surrounding concentric fibrosis (Fan et al., 2012).

Inflammatory Myofibroblastic Tumor (IMT)

IMT are spindle tumors which may form in any body district. In literature, IMT of the bladder has been classified either as inflammatory pseudotumor, pseudosarcoma, inflammatory pseudosarcomatous fibromyxoid tumor, atypical fibromyxoid tumor, atypical myofibroblastic and plasma cell granulomanodular fasciitis, pseudosarcomatous myofibroblastic tumor, and fibromyxoid pseudotumor (Jones et al., 1993; Houben et al., 2007). More recently it has been proposed to identify this lesion as a tumor exhibiting an inflammatory infiltrate, spindle cell proliferation, absence of significant necrosis, cytologic atypia, and abnormal mitotic figures (Netto et al., 1999). Patients mostly present with painless hematuria; additional symptoms include voiding anomalies, abdominal pain, and palpable abdominal mass; less frequent the presence of fever and weight loss. Differential diagnosis with sarcomas may be a problem because of similar histopathologic features (Weidner, 1995). Other minor problems may arise in differential diagnosis from either benign (leiomyoma, solitary fibrous tumors), or malignant lesions (leiomyosarcoma, sarcomatoid carcinoma, embryonal rhabdomyosarcoma). Thus, the most affordable way to characterize the lesion is immunochemistry; IMT spindle cells normally express vimentin and SMA, and rarely desmin (Hussong et al., 1999); more recently, the over-expression of anaplastic lymphoma kinase (ALK), consequent to gene translocations, has been reported as an affordable molecular marker (Rao et al., 2012). A meta-analysis of bladder IMT in the pediatric age group reveals that local excision with or without partial cystectomy is the most preferred treatment option (Houben et al., 2007). Recurrence or metastasis for bladder IMT in children seems not a problem, yet it should be recalled that literature is still inconclusive because of the relatively low number of affected patients (Janik et al., 2003). Its malignant potential is currently unknown, but clinically these tumors are slow growing and generally follow a benign course. IMT etiology is still an issue. Because of its inflammatory nature, some Authors believe that a chronic phlogosis (infection, autoimmune disease) may cause its formation. Others consider it a low-grade mesenchymal malignancy because of its propensity to infiltrate both bladder wall and perivesical tissue, and for the expression of ALK. However, to date no definitive causes had been clearly recognized (Houben et al., 2007). As for the treatment, available literature favors a conservative, partial cystectomy, or local excision if the tumor is too large for complete removal by TUR (Lekas et al., 2008).

Mesonephric and Clear Cell Adenocarcinomas (CCA) of the Female Genital Tract

Mesonephric adenocarcinoma (of mullerian origin) and clear cell adenocarcinoma (of wolffian origin) of the urinary bladder are rare, highly malignant tumors, which may form at any age. Indeed, 30% of patients are children (Merguerian et al., 2007). Although its origin is not completely clear, evidences about its tubular structure and its usual localization - mainly vagina, but also cervix, uterus and salpinx - suggests that it might evolve from developmental remnants of urogenital tract formation. At presentation, usually patients declare vaginal bleeding or mass. It may be difficult to perform a differential diagnosis with embryonal rhabdomyosarcoma since radiographic analysis reveals strikingly similarities (Merguerian et al., 2007); also non-invasive clear cell adenoma should be ruled out during diagnosis. For these cancers the standard treatment is radical excision, radiotherapy, or both (Tazi et al., 2004; Merguerian et al., 2007). CCA may also be a byproduct of maternal diethylstilbestrol (DES) treatment before 18 weeks of gestation; for this group of exposed children, the incidence raises to about 1:1000 (Melnick et al., 1987; Herbst and Anderson, 1990).

Perivascular Epithelioid Cell Neoplasms (PEComas)

PEComas are a family of mesenchymal tumors composed of histologically and immunohistochemically distinctive perivascular epithelioid cells (Folpe, 2002). The family includes angiomyolipoma (AML), clear cell sugar tumor of the lung (CCST), lymphangioleiomyomatosis (LAM), and rarer tumors in other locations. They are rarely malignant, and the few available data seem to suggest a low recurrence for these lesions (Folpe and Kwiatkowski, 2010; Yin et al., 2012). To date, less than 40 pediatric PEComas have been reported in locations different from the bladder (Yang et al., 2012) and only 13 cases affecting the urinary bladder are reported in the English-language literature worldwide, plus two cases whose report is available in Chinese language only. Among those described in English, only one pediatric case is illustrated, affecting a 16 years old girl (Yin et al., 2012). She presented at age 16 with a 3-year history of vague abdominal discomfort; diagnosis was performed by ultrasound imaging but the mass was not removed. Two years later the girl came back with frequent micturition without hematuria or dysuria; the mass was analyzed again by ultrasonography, CT and NMR. Then, the patient underwent transurethral resection of the bladder tumor (TURBT) and bioptic analysis. Notably, this lesion can be confused with clear cell sarcoma of soft tissue (CCSST) and melanoma because of the strong positivity for melanotic markers, especially when neoplastic cells express the S-100 protein (Yin et al., 2012). However, the majority of PEComas (i) show peculiar cellular morphology, (ii) express muscle markers, whereas most melanotic tumors are negative for actin, and (iii) typical CCSST chromosome translocations are absent in this type of lesions (Yin et al., 2012). In the reported case, no recurrence was discovered after 13 months of follow up.

Nephrogenic Adenoma (NA)

Nephrogenic adenoma is a rare, benign lesion of the urinary tract widely considered a metaplastic response to urothelial trauma, infection, immunosuppression or radiation, but it is also frequent in patients with a history of preceding bladder surgery and/or chronic irritation (Heidenreich et al., 1999), such as augmented bladder (Franke et al., 2011). It affects girls more than boys, with a 5:1 ratio (Merguerian et al., 2007). NA is usually shaped as a papillary formation somehow similar to a low grade and low stage TCC (Heidenreich et al., 1999) but also tubulocystic and mixed papillary/tubulocystic patterns had been described; cystic and tubular morphs are less frequent (Kao and Epstain, 2013).

Pediatric patients usually present with hematuria, dysuria and bladder instability, but the final diagnosis relies upon cystoscopy and cytological analysis of bioptic samples. In difficult cases, an immunohistochemical panel consisting of cytokeratin 7, PAX-2, PAX-8, and MUC-1 may be a useful diagnostic tool (Kao et al., 2013). Lesion removal is usually achieved by transurethral resection and follow-up involves both periodic cystoscopy and antibiotic therapy (Heidenreich et al., 1999; Merguerian et al., 2007). Recurrence rates are as high as 80%, with a latency of 4 years (Merguerian et al., 2007). NA may be occasionally associated to other pathologies, such as prune belly syndrome (two pediatric cases reported to date) (Broecker et al., 2011).

Cavernous Hemangioma (CH)

Hemangioma of the bladder is the second most common hemangioma of the urinary tract (Jahn and Nissen, 1991). CH is a hamartoma, a benign mesenchymal neoplasm which grows at the same rate as the surrounding tissues and is composed of tissue elements normally found at that site, yet developing in a disorganized manner. Most bladder hemangiomas are solitary formations of the cavernous type, and are localized on the posterior wall or dome. Also capillary and arteriovenous hemangiomas exist, but they are less frequent (Rosenberg et al., 1973). CH in childhood is unfrequent, with some cases reported as part of a congenital cavernous condition such as Klippel-Trenaunay-Weber syndrome (Hall, 1971). Patients usually present with macroscopic hematuria; although ultrasonography may drive the diagnosis, the final assessment is usually achieved by cystoscopy (Ikeda et al., 2004; Merguerian et al., 2007). The affected region frequently shows hyperactive tissue, thus biopsy and transurethral resections should be avoided for causing potential extensive bleeding; endoscopic resection, which is hemorrhagic and incomplete, has been replaced by yttrium aluminium garnet (YAG) laser coagulation in the treatment of small tumors (Zini et al., 2001; Ishikawa et al., 2003). In case of laser treatment failure (Ikeda et al., 2004) or large CH dimensions (Pratap et al., 2007), partial cystectomy may be a good alternative choice of treatment. Cure is suggested because there is the suspect that, in the long term, at least some of the CH may develop into malignant formations, such as angiosarcoma (Jason et al., 1998). Despite its generally benign prognosis, CH is a potentially life-threatening condition: among complications due to delayed diagnosis, hemorrhagic shock consequent to massive hematuria is possible (Numanoglu and Tatli, 2008).

Teratoma

Teratoma is an encapsulated tumor including cells from more than one (frequently all three) embryonic layers. These neoplasms have been reported to contain hair, teeth, bone and, very rarely, more complex organs or processes. It may be either benign (dermoid cyst) or not. Due to their embryonic nature, teratomas are likely present since birth, but small formations may not be discovered for long times. Dermoid cyst in the urinary bladder are extremely rare - in literature only seven cases are reported, and to our knowledge only one of them affecting an eight years old girl, who was treated by cystoscopy (Misra et al., 1997); for her, no recurrences were found during a four years follow up.

PARAGANGLIOMA/PHEOCHROMOCYTOMA

Bladder paraganglioma derives from chromaffin tissue of the sympathic system. It is exceedingly uncommon in childhood: it has been described so far in about ten patients aged 7-16 years and its estimated prevalence is 0.06% of bladder tumors (De Pasquale et al., 2011).These neoplasms are usually benign lesions, although malignant forms had been described; in this case it has been suggested that resection should reach the bladder serosa in order to fully remove the tumor (Segawa and Osafune, 2005). They show hormonal activity and associated symptomatology is related to the catecholamine production (De Pasquale et al., 2011). Patients may present with episodic hypertension, headache, diaphoresis and palpitation, occasionally related to urination (Mou et al., 2008), and less frequently with macroscopic hematuria and anemia (Bohn et al., 2011). Its treatment is commonly transurethral resection or partial cystectomy, but recently a less invasive endoscopic treatment with synchronization cystostomy has been successfully used (Xiang et al., 2013). Recurrence has been reported in some cases (Bohn et al., 2011).

LYMPHANGIOMA

Lymphangiomas are benign, soft-tissue tumors of lymphatic origin. In this neoplasm, proliferation of lymphatic tissue probably originates from lymphatic vessels that failed to establish connections with the lymphatic system; consequently, these lesions are likely congenital (Wilson et al., 2006). Only three cases of lymphangioma of the bladder have been reported worldwide since 1983; of them, two were in children. The first case was a child presenting with macroscopic painless hematuria (Bolkier et al., 1983); the patient had a large tumor that was treated with partial cystectomy. The second case was an 8 years old girl presented with a terminal hematuria associated with intermitted fever over one week (Niu et al., 2010). The patient was diagnosed by ultrasonography, retrograde urethrography and CT. An open operation was performed, and the mass was removed by partial cystectomy. There was no evidence of recurrence after a follow up of 3 years.

NEUROFIBROMA

A neurofibroma is a benign nerve sheath tumor in the peripheral nervous system. Usually found in individuals with neurofibromatosis type I (NF1), an autosomal dominant genetically inherited disease affecting approximately 1 in 3000 individuals. Neurofibromas rarely manifest in the genitourinary tract; fewer than 70 cases with bladder involvement have been reported to date. Of these, only about 25 cases have occurred in the pediatric population (Cheng et al., 1999). Clinical symptoms include hematuria, irritation and pelvic mass (Cheng et al., 1999). Although very uncommon, neurofibroma has been reported to involve nearly every level of the genitourinary system, the bladder being most often affected (Kaefer et al., 1997). It entails both spinal (pudendal) and autonomic nerves of the bladder wall, including involvement of visceral ganglia. In most cases the lesion is benign, though some neurofibromas may become malignant; however, this occurred only twice, and only in adults (Scheithauer et al., 1999). The treatment of plexiform neurofibroma is complicated by its intrinsic tendency to involve a very high number of branches, or even an entire plexus of nerves, thereby making it difficult or even impossible to obtain a total resection (Kaefer et al., 1997). An even rarer form of this tumor is the plexiform neurofibroma with diffuse ganglioneuromatosis, of which only two cases had been described so far, only one of them involving a child (Scheithauer et al., 2008). The patient was a 6 years old girl with a 6-day course of painless, sterile, gross hematuria, diagnosed by ultrasound imaging, cystoscopy and needle biopsy. The removal was obtained by partial cystectomy.

BC PEDIATRIC EPIDEMIOLOGY AND PATIENT MANAGEMENT

The treatment and management of pediatric BC patients is an highly debated matter. A large part of incongruence comes from the non uniform definition of "young" and "old" patient; consequently, according to some studies, there are no evident differences between the two groups, while in other studies differences exist (Paner et al., 2011). Indeed, "young" patients had been defined in different studies with a cut off age of either 20, 30, 40 or even 45 years. Consequently, a management standard for children affected by BC does not exist. Paner and collaborators (Paner et al., 2011) made a meta-analysis including all published works available in PubMed, dated between 1960 and 2010, and counting all patients aged 40 years or less; then, they further divided patients into three groups, aged 0-20, 20-30 and 30-40 years (one year overlap). They were able to demonstrate that there is a clear decrease in BC incidence in parallel with decreasing age, being the age range 0-20 the less affected (15/282 patients, or 5.3%, of all BC cases under 40 years old). The additional subdivision of the younger group of patients into four subgroups spaced by 5 years further supported this trend, with children aged 0-5 showing an incidence of 1.9% among all BC cases below the age of 20. These data are in good agreement with those reported in the SEER website (see Introduction).

Also the male to female ratio showed an age-related trend, although males are more prone to BC than females in all age intervals. The overall ratio below 40 years is 3.8:1, but below age 20 the ratio is 5.4:1. Moreover, the Authors also noted that a delayed diagnosis is not uncommon, either because of problem underestimation (hematuria interpreted as an output of benign urethrorrhagia, trauma, infection or congenital urologic anomaly) and/or because of a lower inclination to use invasive diagnostic tools, such as a cystoscope (requiring general anesthesia in babies) or irradiation, in so small children. In some reports, it is described a delay of at least one year after first presentation, involving no less than 26% of patients. Despite this, the vast majority of tumors were solitary lesions, multifocal tumors being as low as 6%. Moreover, patients were mostly affected by low grade tumors (73.4% grade 1, none of grade 3).

Interestingly, TCC grade 1 showed a tendency to decrease with increasing age, in favor of grades 2 and 3 - that is to say that adolescents are more prone to TCC grade 2 (more rarely grade 3) and infants are more prone to TCC grade 1. PUNLMPs (having papillary structure and thickened urothelium, but showing normal cytology), which have a relatively high recurrence rate but low progression, turned out to be the most common bladder tumors in the 0-20 age range. In addition, in these young patients, the predominant situation is the presence of superficial and non-invasive neoplasms (94%); indeed, no patient was found with a stage higher than pT3, and none showed metastases or lymph nodes involvement.

As for the outcome, the meta-analysis revealed that, overall (and with the differences highlighted case by case in the preceding sections) in children are low either recurrence (3.4%), progression (1.1%) and death (1.1%), this trend being strikingly different from elder patients aged >20 years.

Differential management of young patients starts from diagnosis. As described throughout these pages, the first symptom is almost always gross hematuria.

The use of diagnostic techniques such as cystoscopy (invasive), bladder mapping (aimless for unifocal lesions), urine cytology (ineffective for low grade tumors), excretory urography (low sensitivity in young patients) and CT (not advised in children because of radiations) are not considered a standard in these patients. Instead, ultrasonography demonstrated very good sensitivity and low invasiveness, thus this technique is generally the elective method for both first-line diagnosis and post-treatment surveillance. Whenever possible, the removal of BC should be nerve-sparing in both sexes, to assure these patients a good quality of life. The aim is hence to preserve sexual function (vagina lubrification for sexual intercourse in females), potency (seminal vesicle conservation in males), fertility (avoiding transaction of efferent ducts and prostate maintenance in males, maintaining uterus in females), normal voiding and complete urinary continence; of course, these options must be evaluated case by case, according to patient conditions and tumor size/localization.

CONCLUSION

BC in young patients, aged 0-20 years, is different from that of elder people. It shows a much lower incidence; presents an higher male to female ratio; it is usually unifocal; it is mainly low grade, low stage and non invasive; does not show a field effect; its genetic/environmental causes are different from those of the adults, and are mostly currently unknown; the outcome is usually favorable; the diagnosis should be performed by minimally invasive methods, using ultrasound imaging whenever achievable; the treatment should, if possible, take care of the long term quality of life of the patient. For all these reasons, despite the obvious similarities, BC in young and old patients (cut-off at 20 years) should be treated as different diseases, thus needing dissimilar management.

REFERENCES

Blasco Casares FJ; Sacristán Sanfelipe J; Ibarz Servio L; Batalla Cadira JL; Ruiz Marcellán FJ. Characteristics of bladder leiomyoma in our setting. *Arch. Esp. Urol.* 1995 Dec;48(10):987-90.

Bolkier M; Ginesin Y; Lichtig C; Levin DR. Lymphangioma of bladder. *J. Urol.* 1983 May;129(5):1049-50.

Brahmi U; Rajwanshi A; Joshi K; Dey P; Vohra H; Ganguly NK; Gupta SK. Automated nuclear image morphometry on fine needle aspiration smears of malignant round cell tumors. *Anal. Quant. Cytol. Histol.* 2001 Aug;23(4):287-90.

Broecker JS; Steelman CK; Broecker BH; Shehata BM. Nephrogenic adenoma of the bladder in a prune belly syndrome patient: case report and review of the literature. *Fetal. Pediatr Pathol.* 2011;30(5):296-300. doi: 10.3109/15513815.2011.572958.

Brucker B; Ernst L; Meadows A; Zderic S. A second leiomyosarcoma in the urinary bladder of a child with a history of retinoblastoma 12 years following partial cystectomy. *Pediatr Blood Cancer.* 2006 Jun;46(7):811-4.

Bujons A; Caffaratti J; Garat JM; Villavicencio H. Long-term follow-up of transitional cell carcinoma of the bladder in childhood. *J. Pediatr Urol.* 2014 Feb;10(1):167-70. doi: 10.1016/j.jpurol.2013.08.002.

Chandy PC; Pai MG; Budihal MR; Kaulgud SR. Carcinoma of bladder in young children: report of 2 cases. *J. Urol.* 1975; 113:264e5.

Chen H; Niu ZB; Yang Y. Bladder leiomyoma in a 6-year-old boy. *Urology.* 2012 Feb;79(2):434-6. doi: 10.1016/j.urology.2011.06.011.

Cheng L; Scheithauer BW; Leibovich BC; Ramnani DM; Cheville JC; Bostwick DG. Neurofibroma of the urinary bladder. *Cancer.* 1999 Aug 1;86(3):505-13.

Chigurupati R; Alfatooni A; Myall RW; Hawkins D; Oda D. Orofacial rhabdomyosarcoma in neonates and young children: a review of literature and management of four cases. *Oral. Oncol.* 2002 Jul;38(5):508-15.

Cornella JL; Larson TR; Lee RA; Magrina JF; Kammerer-Doak D. Leiomyoma of the female urethra and bladder: report of twenty-three patients and review of the literature. *Am. J. Obstet. Gynecol.* 1997 Jun;176(6):1278-85.

Dasgupta R; Rodeberg DA. Update on rhabdomyosarcoma. *Semin Pediatr Surg.* 2012 Feb;21(1):68-78. doi: 10.1053/j.sempedsurg.2011.10.007.

Dénes FT; Duarte RJ; Cristófani LM; Lopes RI. Pediatric Genitourinary Oncology. *Front Pediatr*. 2013 Dec 16;1:48. eCollection 2013.

Di Pierro GB; Gulia C; Cristini C; Fraietta G; Marini L; Grande P; Gentile V; Piergentili R. Bladder cancer: a simple model becomes complex. *Curr. Genomics*. 2012 Aug;13(5):395-415. doi: 10.2174/138920212801619232.

Epstein JI; Amin MB; Reuter VR; Mostofi FK. The World Health Organization/International Society of Urological Pathology consensus classification of urothelial (transitional cell) neoplasms of the urinary bladder. Bladder Consensus Conference Committee. *Am. J. Surg. Pathol.* 1998; 22:1435e48.

Fan R; Grignon DJ; Rhee A; Meldrum KK; Cheng L. Exstrophy polyp is a unique pathology entity. *Pediatr Dev. Pathol.* 2012 Nov-Dec;15(6):471-7. doi: 10.2350/12-03-1167-OA.1.

Filipas D; Fisch M; Stein R; Gutjahr P; Hohenfellner R; Thüroff JW. Rhabdomyosarcoma of the bladder, prostate or vagina: the role of surgery. *BJU Int.* 2004 Jan;93(1):125-9.

Folpe AL; Kwiatkowski DJ. Perivascular epithelioid cell neoplasms: pathology and pathogenesis. *Hum. Pathol.* 2010 Jan;41(1):1-15. doi: 10.1016/j.humpath.2009.05.011.

Folpe AL; McKenney JK; Li Z; Smith SJ; Weiss SW. Clear cell myomelanocytic tumor of the thigh: report of a unique case. *Am. J. Surg. Pathol.* 2002 Jun;26(6):809-12.

Franke EI; Misseri R; Cain MP; Kaefer M; Meldrum KK; Fan R; Rink RC. Nephrogenic adenoma in the augmented bladder. *J. Urol.* 2011 Oct;186(4 Suppl):1586-9. doi: 10.1016/j.juro.2011.04.015.

Furuhashi M; Suganuma N. Recurrent bladder leiomyoma with ovarian steroid hormone receptors. *Urology*. 2002 Mar;167(3):1399-400.

Giedl J; Wild PJ; Stoehr R; Junker K; Boehm S; van Oers JM; Zwarthoff EC; Blaszyk H; Fine SW; Humphrey PA; Dehner LP; Amin MB; Epstein JI; Hartmann A. Urothelial neoplasms in individuals younger than 20 years show very few genetic alterations and have a favourable clinical outcome. *Verh Dtsch Ges. Pathol.* 2006;90:253-63.

Gites RF. Tumours of bladder. Campbell urology, 4th ed. vol. 2. WB Saunders; 1979. p. 1041.

Goluboff ET; O'Toole K; Sawczuk IS. Leiomyoma of bladder: report of case and review of literature. *Urology*. 1994 Feb;43(2):238-41.

Gupta S; Bhaijee F; Harmon EP. Mucinous neoplasm arising in a urachal cyst: a first in the pediatric population. *Urology*. 2014 Feb;83(2):455-6. doi: 10.1016/j.urology.2013.09.034.

Hall BD. Bladder hemangiomas in Klippel-Trenaunay-Weber syndrome. *N. Engl. J. Med.* 1971 Oct 28;285(18):1032-3.

Heidenreich A; Zirbes TK; Wolter S; Engelmann UH. Nephrogenic adenoma: A rare bladder tumor in children. *Eur. Urol.* 1999 Oct;36(4):348-53.

Heinzelmann F; Thorwarth D; Lamprecht U; Kaulich TW; Fuchs J; Seitz G; Ebinger M; Handgretinger R; Bamberg M; Weinmann M. Comparison of different adjuvant radiotherapy approaches in childhood bladder/prostate rhabdomyosarcoma treated with conservative surgery. *Strahlenther Onkol.* 2011 Nov;187(11):715-21. doi: 10.1007/s00066-011-2261-3.

Herbst AL; Anderson D. Clear cell adenocarcinoma of the vagina and cervix secondary to intrauterine exposure to diethylstilbestrol. *Semin Surg. Oncol.* 1990;6(6):343-6.

Hoenig DM; McRae S; Chen SC; Diamond DA; Rabinowitz R; Caldamone AA. Transitional cell carcinoma of the bladder in the pediatric patient. *J. Urol.* 1996 Jul;156(1):203-5.

Houben CH; Chan A; Lee KH; Tam YH; To KF; Cheng W; Yeung CK. Inflammatory myofibroblastic tumor of the bladder in children: what can be expected? *Pediatr Surg. Int.* 2007 Aug;23(8):815-9.

Hussong JW; Brown M; Perkins SL; Dehner LP; Coffin CM. Comparison of DNA ploidy, histologic, and immunohistochemical findings with clinical outcome in inflammatory myofibroblastic tumors. *Mod. Pathol.* 1999 Mar;12(3):279-86.

Ikeda T; Shimamoto K; Tanji N; Ohoka H; Nishio S; Yokoyama M; Ikeda M. Cavernous hemangioma of the urinary bladder in an 8-year-old child. *Int. J. Urol.* 2004 Jun;11(6):429-31.

Ishikawa K; Saitoh M; Chida S. Detection of bladder hemangioma in a child by blood-pool scintigraphy. *Pediatr Radiol.* 2003 Jun;33(6):433-5.

Jahn H; Nissen HM. Haemangioma of the urinary tract: review of the literature. *Br. J. Urol.* 1991 Aug;68(2):113-7.

Janik JS; Janik JP; Lovell MA; Hendrickson RJ; Bensard DD; Greffe BS. Recurrent inflammatory pseudotumors in children. *J. Pediatr Surg.* 2003 Oct;38(10):1491-5.

Jason DE; Timothy MK; Monica CM et al. Angiosarcoma of the bladder: A review. *Urology.* 1998; 52: 778–84.

Javadpour N; Mostofi FK. Primary epithelial tumors of the bladder in the first two decades of life. *J. Urol.* 1969 May;101(5):706-10.

Jones EC; Clement PB; Young RH. Inflammatory pseudotumor of the urinary bladder. A clinicopathological, immunohistochemical, ultrastructural, and flow cytometric study of 13 cases. *Am. J. Surg. Pathol.* 1993 Mar;17(3):264-74.

Kaefer M; Adams MC; Rink RC; Keating MA. Principles in management of complex pediatric genitourinary plexiform neurofibroma. *Urology.* 1997 Jun;49(6):936-40.

Kao CS; Epstein JI. Tubular adenoma of the urinary tract: a newly described entity. *Hum. Pathol.* 2013 Sep;44(9):1890-4. doi: 10.1016/j.humpath. 2013.02.017.

Kao CS; Kum JB; Fan R; Grignon DJ; Eble JN; Idrees MT. Nephrogenic adenomas in pediatric patients: a morphologic and immunohistochemical study of 21 cases. *Pediatr Dev. Pathol.* 2013 Mar-Apr;16(2):80-5. doi: 10.2350/12-10-1261-OA.1.

Kim EE; Valenzuela RF; Kumar AJ; Raney RB; Eftekari F. Imaging and clinical spectrum of rhabdomyosarcoma in children. *Clin. Imaging.* 2000 Sep-Oct;24(5):257-62.

Kim SO; Kwon D; Choi C; Baek HJ; Park K; Ryu SB. A case of spontaneous rupture perforation of leiomyosarcoma in the urachus of a young boy. *Int. J. Urol.* 2007 Oct;14(10):960-2.

Lekas A; Parasi A; Papathomas TG; Papatsoris AG; Mennonna MR; Chrisofos M; Deliveliotis C; Lazaris AC. Pseudosarcomatous myofibroblastic lesion of the urinary bladder: a rare entity posing a diagnostic challenge and therapeutic dilemma. *Diagn Pathol.* 2008 Mar 13;3:11. doi: 10.1186/1746-1596-3-11.

Lerena J; Krauel L; García-Aparicio L; Vallasciani S; Suñol M; Rodó J. Transitional cell carcinoma of the bladder in children and adolescents: six-case series and review of the literature. *J. Pediatr Urol.* 2010 Oct;6(5):481-5. doi: 10.1016/j.jpurol.2009.11.006.

Leuschner I; Harms D; Mattke A; Koscielniak E; Treuner J. Rhabdomyosarcoma of the urinary bladder and vagina: a clinicopathologic study with emphasis on recurrent disease: a report from the Kiel Pediatric Tumor Registry and the German CWS Study. *Am. J. Surg. Pathol.* 2001 Jul;25(7):856-64.

Lott S; Lopez-Beltran A; Montironi R; MacLennan GT; Cheng L. Soft tissue tumors of the urinary bladder Part II: malignant neoplasms. *Hum. Pathol.* 2007 Jul;38(7):963-77.

Madgar I; Goldwasser B; Nativ O; Hanani Y; Jonas P. Long-term followup of patients less than 30 years old with transitional cell carcinoma of bladder. *J. Urol.* 1988 May;139(5):933-4.

Martin SA; Sears DL; Sebo TJ; Lohse CM; Cheville JC. Smooth muscle neoplasms of the urinary bladder: a clinicopathologic comparison of leiomyoma and leiomyosarcoma. *Am. J. Surg. Pathol.* 2002 Mar;26(3):292-300.

Matsushima M; Asakura H; Sakamoto H; Horinaga M; Nakahira Y; Yanaihara H. Leiomyoma of the bladder presenting as acute urinary retention in a female patient: urodynamic analysis of lower urinary tract symptom; a case report. *BMC Urol.* 2010 Aug 4;10:13. doi: 10.1186/1471-2490-10-13.

Melicow MM. Tumours of urinary bladder: a clinico-pathological analysis of over 2500 specimens and biopsies. *J. Urol.* 1955;74:498e521.

Melnick S; Cole P; Anderson D; Herbst A. Rates and risks of diethylstilbestrol-related clear-cell adenocarcinoma of the vagina and cervix. An update. *N. Engl. J. Med.* 1987 Feb 26;316(9):514-6.

Merguerian PA; Cartwright L; Khoury AE. Genitourinary rhabdomyosarcoma and other bladder tumors. In: *The Kelalis–King–Belman Textbook of clinical pediatric urology*, 5th Edition, Docimo, Canning and Khoury Eds. 2007, 969-998.

Misra S; Agarwal PK; Tandon RK; Wakhlu AK; Misra NC. Bladder teratoma: a case report and review of literature. *Indian J. Cancer.* 1997 Mar;34(1):20-1.

Mutchler RW Jr; Gorder JL. Leiomyoma of the bladder in a child. *Br. J. Radiol.* 1972 Jul;45(535):538-40.

Nelson CP; Dunn RL; Wei JT. Contemporary epidemiology of bladder exstrophy in the United States. *J. Urol.* 2005 May;173(5):1728-31.

Netto JM; Pérez LM; Kelly DR; Joseph DB. Pediatric inflammatory bladder tumors: myofibroblastic and eosinophilic subtypes. *J. Urol.* 1999 Oct;162(4):1424-9.

Newton WA Jr; Gehan EA; Webber BL; Marsden HB; van Unnik AJ; Hamoudi AB; Tsokos MG; Shimada H; Harms D; Schmidt D; et al. Classification of rhabdomyosarcomas and related sarcomas. Pathologic aspects and proposal for a new classification--an Intergroup Rhabdomyosarcoma Study. *Cancer.* 1995 Sep 15;76(6):1073-85.

Niu ZB; Yang Y; Hou Y; Chen H; Liu X; Wang CL. Lymphangioma of bladder. *Urology.* 2010 Oct;76(4):955-7. doi: 10.1016/j.urology. 2010.03.050.

Noyes D; Vinson RK. Urachal leiomyosarcoma. *Urology.* 1981 Mar;17(3):279-80.

Numanoğlu KV; Tatli D. A rare cause of hemorrhagic shock in children: bladder hemangioma. *J. Pediatr. Surg.* 2008 Jul;43(7):e1-3. doi: 10.1016/j.jpedsurg.2008.02.057.

Ognjanovic S; Linabery AM; Charbonneau B; Ross JA. Trends in childhood rhabdomyosarcoma incidence and survival in the United States, 1975-2005. *Cancer.* 2009 Sep 15;115(18):4218-26. doi: 10.1002/cncr.24465.

Ozturk U; Goktug HN; Tuygun C; Sener NC; Yesil S; Bakirtas H; Imamoglu MA. Pediatric bladder rhabdomyosarcoma: report of organ sparing treatment of two cases. *J. Pediatr Urol.* 2013 Apr;9(2):e111-3. doi: 10.1016/j.jpurol.2012.11.005.

Paner GP; Zehnder P; Amin AM; Husain AN; Desai MM. Urothelial neoplasms of the urinary bladder occurring in young adult and pediatric patients: a comprehensive review of literature with implications for patient management. *Adv. Anat. Pathol.* 2011 Jan;18(1):79-89. doi: 10.1097/PAP.0b013e318204c0cf.

Parekh DJ; Jung C; O'Conner J; Dutta S; Smith ER Jr. Leiomyosarcoma in urinary bladder after cyclophosphamide therapy for retinoblastoma and review of bladder sarcomas. *Urology.* 2002 Jul;60(1):164.

Paulhac P; Maisonnette F; Bourg S; Dumas JP; Colombeau P. Adenocarcinoma in the exstrophic bladder. *Urology.* 1999 Oct;54(4):744.

Pedersen-Bjergaard J; Jønsson V; Pedersen M; Hou-Jensen K. Leiomyosarcoma of the urinary bladder after cyclophosphamide. *J. Clin. Oncol.* 1995 Feb;13(2):532-3.

Pratap A; Tiwari A; Pandey SR; Agrawal B; Paudel G; Adhikary S; Kumar A. Giant cavernous hemangiolymphangioma of the bladder without cutaneous hemangiomatosis causing massive hematuria in a child. *J. Pediatr. Urol.* 2007 Aug;3(4):326-9. doi: 10.1016/j.jpurol.2006.10.010.

Punyko JA; Mertens AC; Baker KS; Ness KK; Robison LL; Gurney JG. Long-term survival probabilities for childhood rhabdomyosarcoma. A population-based evaluation. *Cancer.* 2005 Apr 1;103(7):1475-83.

Qualman SJ; Coffin CM; Newton WA; Hojo H; Triche TJ; Parham DM; Crist WM. Intergroup Rhabdomyosarcoma Study: update for pathologists. *Pediatr Dev. Pathol.* 1998 Nov-Dec;1(6):550-61.

Rao RN; Ranjan P; Singla N; Pandey R. Inflammatory myofibroblastic tumor of the urinary bladder diagnosed by anaplastic lymphoma kinase immunostaining. *Urol. Ann.* 2012 May;4(2):115-8. doi: 10.4103/0974-7796.95567.

Rosenberg J; Golimbu M; Suarez J; Morales P. Congenital arteriovenous malformation of the bladder. *J. Urol.* 1973 Apr;109(4):605-8.

Ruiz E; Alarcón Caba M; Toselli L; Moldes J; Ormaechea M; de Badiola F; Christiansen S. Transitional cell carcinoma of the bladder in adolescents: a diagnosis to bear in mind. *Arch. Argent Pediatr.* 2009 Feb;107(1):49-52. doi: 10.1590/S0325-00752009000100011.

Savage N; Linn D; McDonough C; Donohoe JM; Franco A; Reuter V; Biddinger PW; Eaton KW; Biegel JA; Sharma S. Molecularly confirmed primary malignant rhabdoid tumor of the urinary bladder: implications of accurate diagnosis. *Ann. Diagn Pathol.* 2012 Dec;16(6):504-7. doi: 10.1016/j.anndiagpath.2011.04.008. Epub 2011 Jul 19.

Scheithauer BW; Santi M; Richter ER; Belman B; Rushing EJ. Diffuse ganglioneuromatosis and plexiform neurofibroma of the urinary bladder: report of a pediatric example and literature review. *Hum. Pathol.* 2008 Nov;39(11):1708-12. doi: 10.1016/j.humpath.2008.02.019.

Scheithauer BW; Woodruff J; Erlandson RA. Neurofibroma (Chapter 8). In: Rosai J, Sobin LH editors. *Atlas of tumor pathology - tumors of the peripheral nervous system*, Third series, Fascicle 24. Washington (DC): Armed Forces Institute of Pathology; 1999. p. 177-218.

Schubert GE; Pavkovic MB; Bethke-Bedürftig BA. Tubular urachal remnants in adult bladders. *J. Urol.* 1982 Jan;127(1):40-2.

Siefker-Radtke A. Urachal adenocarcinoma: a clinician's guide for treatment. *Semin Oncol.* 2012 Oct;39(5):619-24. doi: 10.1053/j. seminoncol. 2012.08.011.

Smeulders N; Woodhouse CR. Neoplasia in adult exstrophy patients. *BJU Int.* 2001 May;87(7):623-8.

Tazi H; Tazi K; Ouali M; Koutani A; Hachimi M; Lakrissa A. Urinary bladder mesonephric clear cell adenocarcinoma. *Prog. Urol.* 2004 Dec;14(6):1209-12.

Teran AZ; Gambrell RD Jr. Leiomyoma of the bladder: case report and review of the literature. *Int J Fertil.* 1989 Jul-Aug;34(4):289-92.

Thomas G; Gera P; Arbuckle S; Cohen R. Transitional cell papilloma of the bladder in a child: a case report and review of literature. *J. Pediatr. Urol.* 2006 Feb;2(1):59-62. doi: 10.1016/j.jpurol.2005.05.009.

Walterhouse D; Watson A. Optimal management strategies for rhabdomyosarcoma in children. *Paediatr Drugs.* 2007;9(6):391-400.

Weidner N. Inflammatory (myofibroblastic) pseudotumor of the bladder: a review and differential diagnosis. *Adv. Anat Pathol.* 1995;2(6):362-375.

Wesche WA; Khare VK; Chesney TM; Jenkins JJ. Non-hematopoietic cutaneous metastases in children and adolescents: thirty years experience at St. Jude Children's Research Hospital. *J. Cutan Pathol.* 2000 Nov;27(10):485-92.

Wilson SR; Bohrer S; Losada R; Price AP. Retroperitoneal lymphangioma: an unusual location and presentation. *J. Pediatr Surg.* 2006 Mar;41(3):603-5.

Wu HY; Snyder HM 3rd; Womer RB. Genitourinary rhabdomyosarcoma: which treatment, how much, and when? *J. Pediatr Urol.* 2009 Dec;5(6):501-6. doi: 10.1016/j.jpurol.2009.06.011.

Yang W; Li G; Wei-qiang Z. Multifocal PEComa (PEComatosis) of the female genital tract and pelvis: a case report and review of the literature. *Diagn Pathol.* 2012 Mar 9;7:23. doi: 10.1186/1746-1596-7-23.

Yin L; Bu H; Chen M; Yu J; Zhuang H; Chen J; Zhang H. Perivascular epithelioid cell neoplasm of the urinary bladder in an adolescent: a case report and review of the literature. *Diagn Pathol.* 2012 Dec 31;7:183. doi: 10.1186/1746-1596-7-183.

Zini L; Amara N; Graziana JP; Villers A; Biserte J; Mazeman E. Klippel-Trenaunay syndrome and multiple vesical hemangiomas: treatment with Neodymium:YAG laser. *Prog. Urol.* 2001 Dec;11(6):1282-4.

In: Bladder Cancer
Editor: Samantha Haggerty
ISBN: 978-1-63321-666-2

Chapter 4

MULTI-TASKING CHEMOINFORMATIC MODEL FOR THE EFFICIENT DISCOVERY OF POTENT AND SAFER ANTI-BLADDER CANCER AGENTS

Alejandro Speck-Planche* and M. N. D. S. Cordeiro
REQUIMTE/Department of Chemistry and Biochemistry,
University of Porto, Porto, Portugal

ABSTRACT

Cancers can be considered as a group of diseases, where cells undergo an uncontrolled growth, and malignant tumors are formed. Between them, bladder cancer (BLC) is an aggressive type of cancer, which can propagate from the urinary bladder to other organs in the human body. BLC is the seventh most common cancer around the world, contributing with more than 4% of all deaths caused by cancers. A very good alternative in the battle against this serious disease is the use of chemotherapy. However, for the design of efficient anti-BLC agents, it is necessary to cover a huge space in terms of molecular diversity and complexity. Consequently, chemoinformatics could be a great ally, helping to rationalize the discovery of new and versatile anti-BLC drugs in terms of diminution of financial resources and time. Current computer-

* To whom correspondence should be addressed: E-mail: alejspivanovich@gmail.com; Fax: +351 220402659 (ASP) E-mail: ncordeir@fc.up.pt; Fax: +351 220402659 (ASP).

aided models are able to predict anti-BLC activity against only one biological target (protein, cancer cell line) by using very limited and homogenous datasets. On the other hand, there is no information related with the possible safety of anti-BLC agents which have been tested. In this chapter, we introduce a multi-tasking (mtk) chemoinformatic model for simultaneous prediction of anti-BLC activity and safety profiles such as ADMET (absorption, distribution, metabolism, elimination, toxicity) properties. At the same time, we provide two useful insights regarding the molecular patterns that can be responsible for the anti-BLC activity and/or ADMET properties. In this sense, we give a physicochemical and/or structural explanation about the molecular descriptors which entered in our mtk-chemoinformatic model, and how a defined biological effect can be enhanced. On the other hand, we show a procedure for the calculation and analysis of quantitative contributions of molecular fragments to the biological effects, which can be a useful guide for experts working in medicinal chemistry and pharmaceutical sciences.

INTRODUCTION

During centuries, mankind has been afflicted by dissimilar dangerous diseases. Among them, cancers have always constituted serious health problems, and their devastating powers have caused a remarkable impact in terms of incidence and mortality. Cancers are characterized by uncontrolled growth and multiplication of cells in different organs, resulting in fatal consequence for humans. A study conducted in countries belonging to the European Union (EU) confirmed more than 930,000 annual deaths due to different types of cancers [1]. One of the classes of cancers which deserve more attention is that associated with the urinary bladder. In this sense, bladder cancer (BLC) remains as one of the most common cancers worldwide, with more than 335,000 new cases each year, being Western Europe, North America, Australia and UK the most affected geographic regions [2]. If we take into consideration all these ideas mentioned above, it is intuitive to deduce that the search for efficacious anti-BLC agents is a tremendous challenge for the scientific community, and the success of this process will depend on two very important aspects: the potent activity of the chemicals in order to eradicate (or at least to diminish) the proliferation of BLC cells, and the safety profile of these chemicals for human health. The development of science and technology has provided the creation of wide-spectrum anti-cancer drugs (Figure 1), which are currently employed alone or in combined chemotherapy against many cancers, including BLC [3-5].

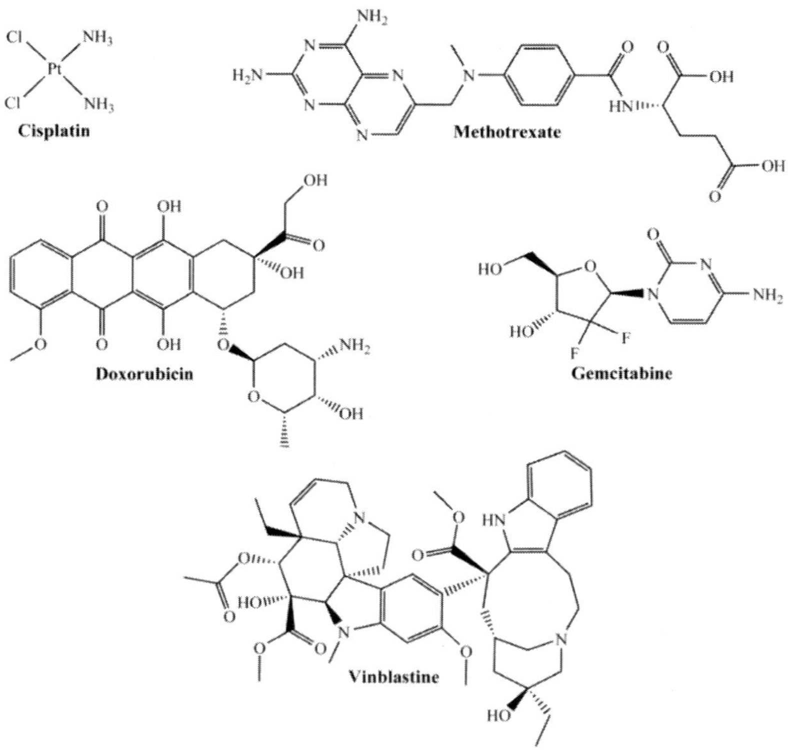

Figure 1. Principal anti-cancer drugs used against BLC.

However, cancer cells have become resistant to many anti-cancer drugs [6]. Although this phenomenon known as anti-neoplastic resistance has multiple explanations, there are very strong arguments from the perspective of drug discovery. For instance, the design of the anti-cancer drugs depicted in Figure 1 (as in the case of many other drugs) has been based on a misconceived strategy of one drug for one target [7], which means that these drugs were developed because of their high affinities to the corresponding (but specific) targets. The appearance of anti-neoplastic resistance obligates the use of 'cocktails' of anti-cancer drugs, increasing the number of adverse effects remarkably. On the other hand, recent advances in systems biology and complexity sciences demonstrate that cancers are multi-factorial in nature [8]. For this reason, current drug discovery strategies that target only one of multiple factors associated to BLC (for example specific inhibitors of proteins) have low probabilities to designing highly efficacious. Novel insights in drug discovery support the fact that multi-target (mt) drugs can offer an advantage over those with 'mono-target' behavior [9]. This comes from the fact that mt-drugs may have a relatively low affinity to different targets, but they remain sufficiently active against several of them. Consequently, mt-drugs might have exhibited a narrower range of side effects than high-affinity mono-target drugs [10]. Another aspect of transcendental importance is the safety of an anti-cancer agent. When any drug candidate is designed, special attention is paid to the presence of desirable ADMET (absorption, distribution, metabolism, excretion, toxicity) parameters [11-12], that represent a major cause for drug approval/disapproval. Drug discovery is a very slow process, which consumes enormous quantity of financial resources and time [13]. For this reason, computer-assisted methods may be needed to rationalize the design of drugs with desired biological activities and safety profiles. In this sense, chemoinformatic models have served as tools to perform virtual search for molecules with dissimilar activities [14-22]. Indeed, in the field of anti-cancer research, many chemoinformatic models have been reported in the last two years [23-33], with only one real promising work in the discovery of anti-BLC agents [34]. We need to emphasize that most chemoinformatic models reported to date have employed very limited datasets of structurally related compounds, where the studies are carried out against only one target (protein, cell line). In any case, there is not model able to predict anti-BLC activities and ADMET parameters simultaneously. The existence of such model would be of great interest, because the rational design of anti-BLC drugs could be guided in different stages, and a deeper understanding of the molecular patterns responsible for the anti-BLC activities and safety profiles could be achieved. Recent evolution in the development of chemoinformatic models has demonstrated the possibility of integrating multiple kinds of chemical and biological data [35-46] with large and heterogeneous dataset of compounds. For this reason, in this chapter, we introduce for the first time, a multi-tasking (mtk) chemoinformatic model for simultaneous prediction of anti-BLC activities and ADMET properties of drugs/chemicals.

MATERIALS AND METHODS

Dataset, Molecular Descriptors and Creation of the Mtk-Chemoinformatic Model

The key steps involved in the construction of mtk-chemoinformatic models have been reported very recently [38, 42-50]. Therefore, we will only mention the fundamental details. The dataset was created by extracting all data from CHEMBL [51], an accurate database which can be found at https://www.ebi.ac.uk/chembl/. Our dataset contained 22648 drugs/chemicals. Taking into consideration that chemicals were tested against more than one experimental condition, we had 39198 cases in total. Thus, at least 1 of 16 measures of biological effects (anti-BLC activities, ADMET properties) was considered, where the assays were carried out against at least 1 of 49 targets (b_t) including BLC cell lines, proteins associated to BLC, laboratory animals, and humans. All the assays contained at least 1 of 8 categories of target mapping (t_m), which defined whether a particular test was linked to specific type of target. We would like to emphasize that the term "experimental condition" should be viewed as an ontology with the form c_j =>(m_e, b_t, t_m). This ontology is also influenced by two external elements. The first of them is p_a, characterizing the priori probability of finding an assay with specific information. Our dataset had assays based on the study of binding (p_a=0.153), functional effects (p_a=0.675) or ADMET processes (p_a=0.172). The second element is p_c, which describes the priori probability of finding an assay with a specific level of curation/reliability. Thus, p_c=0.550 for the category called autocuration (lowest reliability), p_c=0.750 for the category called intermediate, and p_c=1.000 for the category named expert.

Each of the 39198 cases was assigned to 1 of 2 possible classes called "positive" and "negative". These classes were related with the biological effect of a chemical i [$BE_i(c_j)$] in a defined experimental condition c_j. Therefore, any case/chemical was selected as positive [$BE_i(c_j)$=1] if its anti-BLC activity or ADMET property complied with certain cutoff values (Table 1), otherwise, the case was considered as negative [$BE_i(c_j)= -1$]. For the whole dataset, we used a *.txt file containing the SMILES codes of the cases, and with the use of the software MODELAB 1.5 [52], descriptors known as spectral moments of bond adjacency matrix (from order 1 to 6) were calculated [53-55]. These descriptors were weighted by physicochemical properties such as hydrophobicity, polar surface area, polarizability, atomic weight, and the ability of the atoms to act as hydrogen bond acceptors.

We need to point out that the descriptors mentioned above can only consider the chemical structure, but they are not able to contain information regarding the different elements of the ontology c_j (and/or the external factors p_a and p_c) that can be changed. For this reason, we generated new sets of molecular descriptors by applying the moving average approach [56], according to the following expression:

$$D\mu_k(PP)c_j = p_a \cdot p_c \cdot [\mu_k(PP) - AVG\mu_k(PP)c_j] \tag{1}$$

where $\mu_k(PP)$ is the spectral moment of order k of the bond adjacency matrix, weighted by a physicochemical property (PP). On the other hand, $AVG\mu_k(PP)c_j$ characterizes a group n_j of chemicals tested by considering the same element of the ontology c_j. For instance, for the case of b_t, this descriptor was defined as the average of all the $\mu_k(PP)$ values of the chemicals which were assayed by considering the same target. This procedure was applied to each element of the ontology c_j. We only employed the descriptors of type $D\mu_k(PP)c_j$ because they describe both the molecular structure and the combination of different elements in the experimental condition.

The dataset containing 39198 cases was randomly divided into two series: training and prediction sets. The training set was used to construct the mtk-chemoinformatic model, being comprised by 29441 cases, 13255 of them assigned to the class of positive and 16186 considered as negative. The prediction (validation) set was used to demonstrate the predictive power of the model. This set was formed by 9757 cases, 4344 positive and 5413 negative. Cases in prediction set were never used in the training set. We employed linear discriminant analysis (LDA) as pattern classification technique in order to search for the best model, and the software STATISTICA [57] was used to perform this task. Forward stepwise procedure was used as variable selection strategy. The mtk-chemoinformatic model can be represented by the following expression:

$$BE_i(c_j) = a_0 + \sum b_i \cdot D\mu_k(PP)c_j \tag{2}$$

where $BE_i(c_j)$ is the real score predicting the propensity of a compound to have a defined biological effect under a defined experimental condition. The term a_0 is the constant, while b_i represents the different coefficients of the molecular descriptors. We assessed the statistical quality and predictive power of the model by analyzing different indices such as Wilks' lambda (λ), the chi-square (χ^2), and p-level [56]. We determined the percentages of correct classification for positive (sensitivity), negative (specificity), and overall classification, as well as Mathew's correlation coefficients (MCC) [58], and the areas under the ROC (receiver operating characteristic) curves [59]. All these statistical indices were calculated for both training and prediction sets.

Table 1. Cutoff values for the conditions to consider a case as positive

Measure of effect (Units)[a]	Biological Profile	Concept	Cutoff
AC_{50} (nM)	ADMET (Metabolism)	Concentration to elicit the 50% of the maximal effect	≤6309.58
AUC (μM.hr)iv-LA	ADMET (Bioavailability, elimination)	Area under the curve after intravenous administration in laboratory animals (*Mus musculus* and/or *Rattus norvegicus*)	≥10.04
AUC (μM.hr)oral-H	ADMET (Bioavailability, elimination)	Area under the curve after oral administration in humans	≥31.19
AUC (μM.hr)oral-LA	ADMET (Bioavailability, elimination)	Area under the curve after oral administration in laboratory animals (*Mus musculus* and/or *Rattus norvegicus*)	≥15.00
F (%)oral	ADMET (Bioavailability)	Oral bioavailability assessed as the fraction of an oral administered drug that reaches systemic circulation	≥50.00
IC_{50} (nM)	Anti-BLC activity	Concentration required to inhibit 50% of the growth of any BLC cell line	≤10000.00
IC_{50} (nM)ip	Anti-BLC activity	Concentration required to inhibit 50% of the activity of any protein/enzyme associated to BLC	≤200.00
Ki (nM)ip	Anti-BLC activity	Inhibition constant associated to a protein/enzyme present in BLC	≤161.00
LD_{50} (μmol/kg)ip	ADMET (Toxicity)	Lethal dose at 50% after intraperitoneal administration	≥390.00
LD_{50} (μmol/kg)oral	ADMET (Toxicity)	Lethal dose at 50% after oral administration	≥1060.00
Papp (nm/s)	ADMET (Absorption)	Permeability	≥200.00
PPB (%)	ADMET (Distribution)	Plasma protein binding	≤87.00
$T_{1/2}$ (hr)iv-LA	ADMET (Elimination)	Half life after intravenous administration in laboratory animals (*Mus musculus* and/or *Rattus norvegicus*)	≥0.80
$T_{1/2}$ (hr)oral-H	ADMET (Elimination)	Half life after oral administration in humans	≥3.60
$T_{1/2}$ (hr)oral-LA	ADMET (Elimination)	Half life after oral administration in laboratory animals (*Mus musculus* and/or *Rattus norvegicus*)	≥1.20
Vdss (L/kg)iv	ADMET (Distribution)	Volume of distribution at steady state after intravenous administration	≥0.50

[a] Referred to the element m_e of the ontology c_j.

RESULTS AND DISCUSSION

Mtk-Chemoinformatic Model

The search for the best mtk-chemoinformatic model was conditioned not only by the use of the variable selection strategy, but also, by the principle of parsimony. According to this idea, we chose the model with the highest statistical quality, but containing as few molecular descriptors as possible. Thus, the model contained 8 variables:

$$\begin{aligned} BE_i(c_j) = & -2.778D\mu_1(Hyd)m_e + 4.468\cdot 10^{-4} D\mu_6(Pol)m_e \\ & -2.324\cdot 10^{-3} D\mu_2(PSA)b_t + 0.348D\mu_2(Pol)b_t \\ & +1.002\cdot 10^{-3} D\mu_2(Ato)b_t - 4.492\cdot 10^{-3} D\mu_6(Hyd)t_m \\ & -1.146\cdot 10^{-11} D\mu_6(Ato)t_m - 11.071D\mu_1(Ab - sumB2H)t_m \\ & -0.601 \end{aligned}$$

$$N = 29441 \quad \lambda = 0.474 \quad \chi^2 = 21985.23 \quad p - level < 10^{-16} \tag{3}$$

In Eq. 3, the large χ^2, as well as the small values for the indices λ and p-level indicate the very good statistical quality of our mtk-chemoinformatic, which was able to classify 28164 of 29441 cases (accuracy of 95.66%) in the training set, and 9312 of 9757 cases in the prediction set (95.44%). At the same time, in Table 2, there is a compilation of different statistical indices which supports the idea regarding the great performance of the model. Thus, sensitivity and specificity have values higher than 95% for both, training and prediction sets. On the other hand, the analysis of MCC values demonstrates that there is a remarkable correlation between the observed and predicted values of biological effects. This comes from the fact that MCC is a measure of the quality of binary classifications [58]. As final evidence of the quality and predictive power of the model, we determined the areas under the ROC curves (Figure 2). The value of area was 0.992 for both, training and prediction sets, indicating that our mtk-chemoinformatic model is not a random classifier (area=0.5).

More relevant details about the biological and chemical data associated to each case/chemical, together with the corresponding classifications for all the cases can be found in Supplementary Material 1 file (upon request to the authors).

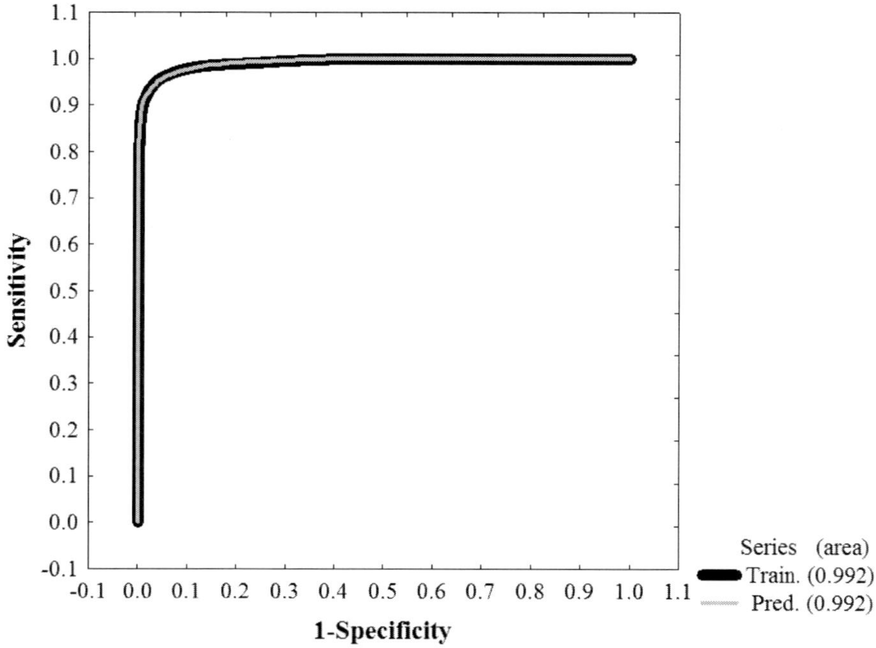

Figure 2. ROC curves obtained for the mtk-chemoinformatic model.

Table 2. Results of classification

Classification	Training set		Prediction set	
	Positive	Negative	Positive	Negative
Total	13255	16186	4344	5413
Correct[a]	12724	15440	4144	5168
Wrong	531	746	200	245
Correct (%)[b]	95.99	95.39	95.40	95.47
Wrong (%)	4.01	4.61	4.60	4.53
MCC	0.913		0.908	

[a] Compounds/cases which were correctly classified by the mtk-chemoinformatic model. [b] Known as sensitivity for positive cases and specificity for negative.

Also, the molecular descriptors of type $AVG\mu_k(PP)c_j$ [used to calculate $D\mu_k(PP)c_j$] appear represented in Supplementary Material 2 file (upon request to the authors).

Table 3. Anti-BLC drugs classified by the mtk-chemoinformatic model

Drug[a]	m_e	b_t	t_m	p_a	p_c	$BE_i(c_j)$[b]	Set	Prob.%[c]
Doxorubicin	IC_{50} (nM)	5637	Cell	0.675	1.000	1	Training	85.05
	IC_{50} (nM)	5637	Cell	0.675	0.750	1	Training	77.63
	IC_{50} (nM)	T-24	Cell	0.675	0.750	1	Training	98.81
	IC_{50} (nM)	J82	Cell	0.675	0.550	1	Training	71.28
	IC_{50} (nM)	5637	Cell	0.675	0.550	1	Training	69.97
	IC_{50} (nM)	T-24	Cell	0.675	0.550	1	Prediction	95.98
	IC_{50} (nM)	SW780	Cell	0.675	0.550	-1	Training	88.33
	IC_{50} (nM)ip	ERBB2	Protein	0.153	0.550	-1	Training	65.36
	Vdss (L/kg)iv	*Homo sapiens*	Animal	0.172	0.550	1	Training	57.59
Vinblastine	IC_{50} (nM)	5637	Cell	0.675	0.550	1	Training	55.19
	IC_{50} (nM)	T-24	Cell	0.675	0.550	1	Prediction	92.67
	IC_{50} (nM)	J82	Cell	0.675	0.550	1	Prediction	56.75
	Vdss (L/kg)iv	*Homo sapiens*	Animal	0.172	0.550	1	Prediction	53.65
Methotrexate	F (%)oral	*Homo sapiens*	Animal	0.172	0.550	1	Training	59.83
	F (%)oral	*Homo sapiens*	Animal	0.172	0.750	1	Prediction	65.20
	IC_{50} (nM)	5637	Cell	0.675	0.550	1	Training	71.88
	IC_{50} (nM)	J82	Cell	0.675	0.550	1	Training	73.14
Gemcitabine	IC_{50} (nM)	KU-19-19	Cell	0.675	0.550	-1	Prediction	99.79
	IC_{50} (nM)	SW780	Cell	0.675	0.550	-1	Training	99.97

[a] This table represents a summary of multiple predictions performed by the mtk-chemoinformatic model. Such predictions were realized against different anti-BLC drugs which were reported in our dataset. [b] Assignations realized for the anti-BLC drugs according to the cutoff values of biological effects represented in Table 1. [c] Probability of the drug to be classified according to its observed value of biological effect [$BE_i(c_j)$].

If we consider all the statistical indices reported here, as well as the diverse experimental conditions under which the chemicals were tested (Materials & Methods), we can conclude that the mtk-chemoinformatic model is a promising tool to perform virtual screening of potent and safer anti-BLC agents, and its statistical quality and predictive power is comparable with other models created in the literature [35-46]. Indeed, in Table 3, there is a summary of the classifications for different biological effects (anti-BLC activities and ADMET parameters), which were realized by our mtk-chemoinformatic model, and where the principal anti-BLC drugs reported in our dataset have been correctly identified 100% of the times. For instance, doxorubicin was reported 9 times in our dataset, and the mtk-chemoinformatic model could correctly assess that this drug is very active against different BLC cell lines, inactive against the protein ERBB2, and had an excellent volume distribution at steady state. Similar analyses were made for the other anti-BLC drugs.

Physicochemical Interpretation of the Molecular Descriptors

When any chemoinformatic model is created, only the best descriptors are selected. The objective is to achieve a clearer characterization of the information associated to the changes of the biological effects of the compounds, as results of the corresponding variations in their chemical structures. In any case, there is a tendency in the construction of prospective chemoinformatic models, i.e., those models which can be used as tools to perform virtual screening of large and heterogeneous databases of molecules. The goal of the prospective predictions is to speed up the search of new and potent pharmacological activities as well as desirable safety profiles [15-22, 35-46]. However, the abuse of the concept of prospective predictions has turned the current chemoinformatic models into "black boxes", where the analyst enters a huge (and sometimes indiscriminate) set of data, and the results of the predictions are obtained according to certain criteria. In those cases where the model is based on classification tasks, the analyst will never know why a chemical was classified to belong to one group or another, because there will be no information regarding the molecular patterns responsible for the presence or absence of a defined biological effect. This comes from the fact that the physicochemical interpretations of the molecular descriptors in the model are usually underestimated or omitted.

In our opinion, the physicochemical interpretation of each molecular descriptor in a model is an element of particular importance. In this chapter, we have developed an mtk-chemoinformatic model with an excellent performance, and one of its advantages is that the molecular descriptors depicted in Eq. 3 have simple physicochemical and/or structural interpretations. First of all, we would like to emphasize that all the descriptors in our mtk-chemoinformatic model depend on the molecular structure and the elements of the ontology c_j, and they will be also influenced by the priori probabilities p_a and p_c. However, due to the fact that these priori probabilities remain constant for a defined experimental condition, we will only be focused on the elements of the ontology c_j. All the explanations in this subsection of the book chapter will be devoted to explain how the different molecular descriptors can vary in order to enhance/increase the biological effect under a defined experimental condition.

For instance, $D\mu_1(Hyd)m_e$ describes the decrease in the global hydrophobicity of the molecule, depending on the chemical structure and the measure of biological effect. A similar tendency in the diminution of the hydrophobicity is accounted by $D\mu_6(Hyd)t_m$, which characterizes both, the structure of the molecules and the target mapping. For the case of this descriptor, the hydrophobicity should decrease in those regions where there are six-membered cycles and/or 6 bonds (or less) between any two atoms. We need to say that $D\mu_1(Hyd)m_e$ as well as $D\mu_6(Hyd)t_m$ are telling us about the necessary existence of hydrophilic (polar regions) in the molecules. In fact, the presence of hydrophilic regions in the molecules is explained by the descriptor $D\mu_1(Ab\text{-}sumB2H)t_m$, where atoms able to act as hydrogen bond acceptors are considered. Thus, $D\mu_1(Ab\text{-}sumB2H)t_m$ will depend on the molecular structure and the target mapping. Another interesting descriptor is $D\mu_6(Pol)m_e$, that expresses the increment of the polarizability in regions where there are six-membered cycles and/or 6 bonds (or less) between any two atoms. Thus, $D\mu_6(Pol)m_e$ considers both, the chemical structure and the measure of biological effect. A convergence effect in terms of the increase in the polarizability is described by $D\mu_2(Pol)b_t$, characterizing the structure of the molecule and the biological target, and considering those regions formed by two bonds. In the same molecular regions defined by $D\mu_2(Pol)b_t$, the polar surface area should be decreased, while the atomic weight should be increased. These two properties are accounted by the descriptors $D\mu_2(PSA)b_t$ and $D\mu_2(Ato)b_t$, which have the same dependence as $D\mu_2(Pol)b_t$. In any case, the effect of the atomic weight considered by $D\mu_2(Ato)b_t$ is constrained by $D\mu_6(Ato)t_m$, which depends on the chemical structure and the target mapping, governing the decrease of the atomic weight in those regions where there are six-membered cycles and/or 6 bonds (or less) between any two atoms.

Quantitative Contributions of Fragments to the Biological Effects

Another remarkable and very useful property of our mtk-chemoinformatic model is that all the molecular descriptors comply with the rule of linear additivity, which means that they can be expressed as linear combinations of the number of times in which a fragment appears in any chemical structure [53-55]. This interesting property of the descriptors which entered in the model represented by Eq. 3 allows us to calculate the quantitative contributions of any fragment to diverse biological effects under study [15, 60]. Consequently, it is possible to have a deeper understanding about the relative influence of the dissimilar molecular patterns in the appearance and/or enhancement of any biological effect. We need to point out that the concept "quantitative contributions" is not new, and has demonstrated to be a very useful tool to medicinal and pharmaceutical chemists, because 2D pharmacophores can be automatically generated [15]. If we take into consideration that our model integrates anti-BLC activities with ADMET profiles, then, the calculations of quantitative contributions could serve for the detection of pharmacophores, toxicophores, metabolophores, etc.

In order to show how our mtk-chemoinformatic model works for the calculation of quantitative contributions, we selected 20 molecular fragments (Figure 3). These fragments appear in different chemicals in our dataset. The procedure to perform such calculation has been recently described [50]. Thus, we calculated descriptors of type $\mu_k(PP)$ for each fragment, the values of $D\mu_k(PP)c_j$ for the different experimental conditions were obtained by using the Eq. 1. Then, the values for $D\mu_k(PP)c_j$ were substituted in Eq. 3 in order to calculate the scores of biological effects. For each fragment, the score was divided by the number of links (bonds without considering their multiplicities) in order to eliminate any dependence on the size. Finally, all the scores were standardized, which means that we calculated the difference between the score of biological effect and the total average, and the result was divided by the standard deviation. This last operation has been proposed by some researchers as a way to provide a better interpretation of the quantitative contributions [37].

For each fragments, 474 different quantitative contributions were calculated. This comes from the fact that 474 unique experimental conditions were used. All data regarding the calculation of the aforementioned contributions can be found in Supplementary Material 3 file (upon request to the authors), while a summary can be found in Table 4 and Table 5.

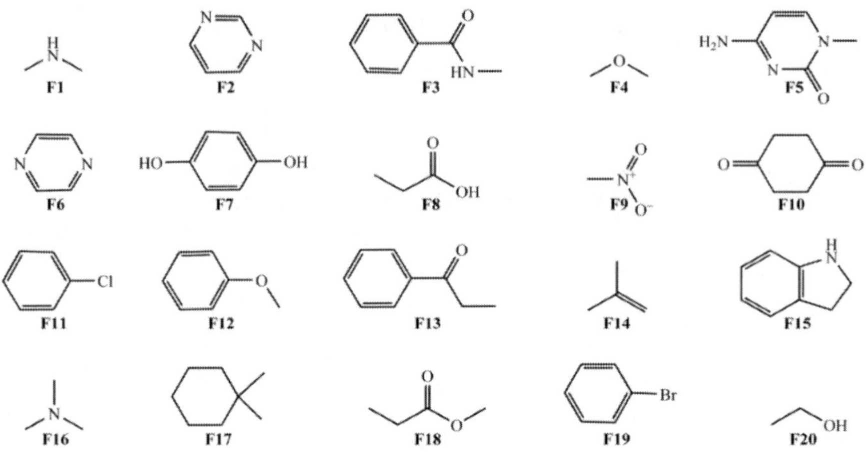

Figure 3. Chemical structures of different molecular fragments.

Table 4. Combination of different elements to form dissimilar experimental conditions

c_j[a,b]	m_e	b_t	t_m	p_a
c_1	AC_{50} (nM)	CYP3A4	Homologous protein	0.675
c_2	AUC (μM.hr)oral-H	Homo sapiens	Animal	0.172
c_3	IC_{50} (nM)	J82	Cell	0.675
c_4	IC_{50} (nM)	KU-19-19	Cell	0.675
c_5	IC_{50} (nM)ip	AKT3	Protein	0.153
c_6	IC_{50} (nM)ip	mTOR	Protein	0.153
c_7	LD_{50} (μmol/kg)oral	Mus musculus	Animal	0.172
c_8	Papp (nm/s)	CHEMBL614058	Cell	0.675
c_9	$T_{1/2}$ (hr)oral-H	Homo sapiens	Animal	0.172
c_{10}	Vdss (L/kg)iv	Homo sapiens	Animal	0.172

[a] The symbol c_j represents the ontology/experimental condition as result of the combination of the elements m_e, b_t, t_m and p_a. [b] The level of curation for all the experimental conditions has the label called expert (p_c=1.000).

If we observe the tables mentioned above, it is intuitive to see that fragments such as F3, F11 to F13, F15, and F19 are the most desirable because of their positive contributions with respect to all the experimental conditions. Accordingly, these fragments could be in principle used for future design of potent and safer anti-BLC agents. Other fragments such as F7 and F10 may be also considered. Notice that some of these fragments mentioned until now appear in the principal anti-cancer drugs which have been represented in Figure 1. For instance, methotrexate contains the fragment F3, doxorubicin has F7, F10, and F12, while vinblastine exhibits F12 and F15 in its structure. On the other hand, fragments such as Fl, F4, and F20 can be viewed as undesirable because of their negative contributions.

Table 5. Quantitative contributions of different fragments to diverse biological effects

Contrib.[a]	c_1	c_2	c_3	c_4	c_5	c_6	c_7	c_8	c_9	c_{10}
F1	-4.895	-0.333	-2.901	-3.733	-0.389	-0.580	-0.116	-4.745	-0.178	-0.215
F2	-0.510	0.521	0.155	-0.122	0.484	0.420	0.593	-0.460	0.572	0.560
F3	0.114	0.627	0.513	0.346	0.601	0.562	0.670	0.144	0.658	0.650
F4	-4.084	-0.126	-2.090	-2.922	-0.205	-0.396	0.091	-3.934	0.029	-0.008
F5	-0.367	0.513	0.076	-0.109	0.496	0.453	0.561	-0.334	0.547	0.539
F6	-0.484	0.527	0.180	-0.097	0.489	0.426	0.600	-0.434	0.579	0.566
F7	-0.240	0.557	0.259	0.051	0.530	0.482	0.611	-0.202	0.595	0.586
F8	-1.705	0.282	-0.709	-1.125	0.243	0.147	0.391	-1.630	0.359	0.341
F9	-2.011	0.271	-0.681	-1.236	0.205	0.077	0.415	-1.911	0.374	0.349
F10	-0.228	0.560	0.270	0.062	0.532	0.484	0.614	-0.191	0.598	0.589
F11	0.243	0.694	0.813	0.575	0.646	0.591	0.756	0.286	0.738	0.728
F12	0.013	0.621	0.511	0.303	0.587	0.539	0.675	0.050	0.660	0.650
F13	0.171	0.642	0.570	0.404	0.614	0.575	0.685	0.201	0.672	0.665
F14	-2.034	0.265	-0.704	-1.259	0.199	0.072	0.409	-1.933	0.368	0.343
F15	0.147	0.635	0.545	0.379	0.608	0.570	0.679	0.177	0.666	0.659
F16	-2.983	0.023	-1.654	-2.208	-0.016	-0.144	0.167	-2.883	0.126	0.101
F17	-0.711	0.436	-0.213	-0.421	0.423	0.375	0.491	-0.674	0.475	0.466
F18	-1.128	0.390	-0.331	-0.664	0.356	0.279	0.476	-1.068	0.451	0.437
F19	0.608	0.787	1.177	0.939	0.729	0.674	0.849	0.650	0.831	0.821
F20	-4.730	-0.291	-2.737	-3.569	-0.351	-0.543	-0.074	-4.580	-0.136	-0.173

[a] As referred in Table 4.

There are two aspects that deserve special attention. First, for the sake of simplicity, we have selected only 20 molecular fragments because our purpose here is to give an idea about how to calculate and interpret the quantitative contributions of the fragments to the biological effects.

But without doubts, a very large number of fragments should be generated and their contributions in different experimental conditions should be determined. The second aspect is that in our dataset, molecules which were assigned to the group of positive can contain fragments with negative contributions. At the same time, molecules considered as negative can have fragments with positive contributions. For this reason, the presence or absence of certain fragments is not a sufficient element for the appearance and/or enhancement of a biological effect. Only the combination and interconnection of the different fragment will define if a chemical will have or not a specific biological effect.

CONCLUSION AND FUTURE PERSPECTIVES

Modern societies have been witnesses of the devastating power of BLC. Novel and efficient chemotherapies are urgently needed to halt this dangerous disease. In this book chapter, the creation of an mtk-chemoinformatic model has been an attempt to provide a computer-assisted tool to rationally complement the experimental techniques in drug discovery. Our model, which was constructed from a large and heterogeneous dataset of chemicals, permitted us to obtain more precise and realistic results by classifying thousands of molecular entities under dissimilar experimental conditions. By combining the physicochemical interpretation of the molecular descriptors with the calculation of quantitative contributions of fragments to the biological effects, an encouraging horizon can be seen: fast and accurate screening of large libraries of fragments.

The present chemoinformatic approach can be extended to other type of cancers, and in the case of BLC, other data such as the occurrence of side effect may be considered. To date, this is the first model which may guide the discovery of potent and safer anti-BLC agent through different stages: from *in vitro* assays to preclinical and clinical trials.

ACKNOWLEDGMENTS

This work is supported by grant No. Pest-C/EQB/LA0006/2011 financed by the Portuguese FCT – *Fundação para a Ciência e a Tecnologia*. A. Speck-Planche acknowledges also FCT and the European Social Fund for financial support (SFRH/BD/77690/2011).

REFERENCES

[1] Lokeshwar, V.B.; Merseburger, A.S.; Hautmann, S.H. *Bladder Tumors: Molecular Aspects and Clinical Management*, Humana Press, Springer Science+Business Media, LLC: New York, Dordrecht, Heidelberg, London, 2011.

[2] MacVicar, D. *Carcinoma of the Bladder*, Cambridge University Press: Cambridge, New York, Melbourne, Madrid, Cape Town, Singapore, São Paulo, 2008.

[3] von der Maase, H. Current and future perspectives in advanced bladder cancer: is there a new standard? *Semin. Oncol.*, 2002, *29*, 3-14.

[4] von der Maase, H.; Sengelov, L.; Roberts, J.T.; Ricci, S.; Dogliotti, L.; Oliver, T.; Moore, M.J.; Zimmermann, A.; Arning, M. Long-term survival results of a randomized trial comparing gemcitabine plus cisplatin, with methotrexate, vinblastine, doxorubicin, plus cisplatin in patients with bladder cancer. *J. Clin. Oncol.*, 2005, *23*, 4602-4608.

[5] Ardavanis, A.; Tryfonopoulos, D.; Alexopoulos, A.; Kandylis, C.; Lainakis, G.; Rigatos, G. Gemcitabine and docetaxel as first-line treatment for advanced urothelial carcinoma: a phase II study. *Br. J. Cancer,* 2005, *92*, 645-650.

[6] Gottesman, M.M. Mechanisms of cancer drug resistance. *Annu. Rev. Med.*, 2002, *53*, 615-627.

[7] Hopkins, A.L. Network pharmacology. *Nat. Biotechnol.*, 2007, *25*, 1110-1111.

[8] Gonzalez-Diaz, H.; Munteanu, C.R. *Topological Indices for Medicinal Chemistry, Biology, Parasitology, Neurological and Social Networks*, Transworld Research Network: Kerala, 2010.

[9] Korcsmáros, T.; Szalay, M.S.; Böde, C.; Kovács, I.A.; Csermely, P. How to design multi-target drugs: target search options in cellular networks. *Expert Opin. Drug Discov.*, 2007, *2*, 1-10.

[10] Csermely, P.; Agoston, V.; Pongor, S. The efficiency of multi-target drugs: the network approach might help drug design. *Trends Pharmacol. Sci.,* 2005, *26*, 178-182.

[11] Borchardt, R.T.; Kerns, E.H.; Hageman, M.J.; Thakker, D.R.; Stevens, J.L. *Optimizing the "Drug-Like" Properties of Leads in Drug Discovery.* Springer Science+Business Media, LLC: New York, NY, 2006; Vol. IV.

[12] Hau, J.; Schapiro, S.J. *Handbook of Laboratory Animal Science: Essential Principles and Practices*, 3rd ed.; CRC Press, Taylor & Francis Group, LLC: Boca Raton, FL, 2011.

[13] Paul, S.M.; Mytelka, D.S.; Dunwiddie, C.T.; Persinger, C.C.; Munos, B.H.; Lindborg, S.R.; Schacht, A.L. How to improve R&D productivity: the pharmaceutical industry's grand challenge. *Nat. Rev. Drug Discov.,* 2010, *9*, 203-214.

[14] Todeschini, R.; Consonni, V. *Molecular Descriptors for Chemoinformatics*, WILEY-VCH Verlag GmbH & Co. KGaA: Weinheim, 2009.

[15] Estrada, E.; Uriarte, E.; Montero, A.; Teijeira, M.; Santana, L.; De Clercq, E. A novel approach for the virtual screening and rational design of anticancer compounds. *J. Med. Chem.,* 2000, *43*, 1975-1985.

[16] Estrada, E.; Vilar, S.; Uriarte, E.; Gutierrez, Y. In silico studies toward the discovery of new anti-HIV nucleoside compounds with the use of TOPS-MODE and 2D/3D connectivity indices. 1. Pyrimidyl derivatives. *J. Chem. Inf. Comput. Sci.,* 2002, *42*, 1194-1203.

[17] Marrero-Ponce, Y.; Castillo-Garit, J.A. 3D-chiral atom, atom-type, and total non-stochastic and stochastic molecular linear indices and their applications to central chirality codification. *J. Comput. Aided Mol. Des.,* 2005, *19*, 369-383.

[18] Casanola-Martin, G.M.; Marrero-Ponce, Y.; Tareq Hassan Khan, M.; Torrens, F.; Perez-Gimenez, F.; Rescigno, A. Atom- and bond-based 2D TOMOCOMD-CARDD approach and ligand-based virtual screening for the drug discovery of new tyrosinase inhibitors. *J. Biomol. Screen.,* 2008, *13*, 1014-1024.

[19] Garcia-Garcia, A.; Galvez, J.; de Julian-Ortiz, J.V.; Garcia-Domenech, R.; Munoz, C.; Guna, R.; Borras, R. Search of chemical scaffolds for novel antituberculosis agents. *J. Biomol. Screen.,* 2005, *10*, 206-214.

[20] Gonzalez-Diaz, H.; Olazabal, E.; Santana, L.; Uriarte, E.; Gonzalez-Diaz, Y.; Castanedo, N. QSAR study of anticoccidial activity for diverse chemical compounds: prediction and experimental assay of trans-2-(2-nitrovinyl)furan. *Bioorg. Med. Chem.,* 2007, *15*, 962-968.

[21] Santana, L.; Gonzalez-Diaz, H.; Quezada, E.; Uriarte, E.; Yanez, M.; Vina, D.; Orallo, F. Quantitative structure-activity relationship and complex network approach to monoamine oxidase A and B inhibitors. *J. Med. Chem.,* 2008, *51*, 6740-6751.

[22] Meneses-Marcel, A.; Rivera-Borroto, O.M.; Marrero-Ponce, Y.; Montero, A.; Machado Tugores, Y.; Escario, J.A.; Gomez Barrio, A.; Montero Pereira, D.; Nogal, J.J.; Kouznetsov, V.V.; Ochoa Puentes, C.; Bohorquez, A.R.; Grau, R.; Torrens, F.; Ibarra-Velarde, F.; Aran, V.J. New antitrichomonal drug-like chemicals selected by bond (edge)-based TOMOCOMD-CARDD descriptors. *J. Biomol. Screen.,* 2008, *13*, 785-794.

[23] Ballante, F.; Caroli, A.; Wickersham, R.B., 3rd; Ragno, R. Hsp90 inhibitors, part 1: definition of 3-D QSAutogrid/R models as a tool for virtual screening. *J. Chem. Inf. Model.,* 2014, *54*, 956-969.

[24] Caroli, A.; Ballante, F.; Wickersham, R.B., 3rd; Corelli, F.; Ragno, R. Hsp90 inhibitors, part 2: combining ligand-based and structure-based approaches for virtual screening application. *J. Chem. Inf. Model.,* 2014, *54*, 970-977.

[25] Kalani, K.; Yadav, D.K.; Singh, A.; Khan, F.; Godbole, M.M.; Srivastava, S.K. QSAR guided semi-synthesis and in-vitro validation of anticancer activity in ursolic acid derivatives. *Curr. Top. Med. Chem.,* 2014, *14*, 1005-1013.

[26] Wu, X.; Zeng, H.; Zhu, X.; Ma, Q.; Hou, Y. Novel pyrrolopyridinone derivatives as anticancer inhibitors towards Cdc7: QSAR studies based on dockings by solvation score approach. *Eur. J. Pharm. Sci.,* 2013, *50*, 323-334.

[27] Jia, J.; Xu, X.; Liu, F.; Guo, X.; Zhang, M.; Lu, M.; Xu, L.; Wei, J.; Zhu, J.; Zhang, S.; Sun, H.; You, Q. Identification, design and bio-evaluation of novel Hsp90 inhibitors by ligand-based virtual screening. *PLoS One,* 2013, *8*, e59315.

[28] Prakash, O.; Khan, F. Cluster based SVR-QSAR modelling for HTS records: an implementation for anticancer leads against human breast cancer. *Comb. Chem. High Throughput Screen.,* 2013, *16*, 511-521.

[29] Prakash, O.; Khan, F. Development of method for three-point data estimation and SVR-QSAR model to screen anti cancer leads. *Comb. Chem. High Throughput Screen.,* 2013, *16*, 425-434.

[30] Yang, W.; Hu, Y.; Yang, Y.S.; Zhang, F.; Zhang, Y.B.; Wang, X.L.; Tang, J.F.; Zhong, W.Q.; Zhu, H.L. Design, modification and 3D QSAR studies of novel naphthalin-containing pyrazoline derivatives

with/without thiourea skeleton as anticancer agents. *Bioorg. Med. Chem.,* 2013, *21*, 1050-1063.

[31] Choi, E.; Lee, C.; Cho, M.; Seo, J.J.; Yang, J.S.; Oh, S.J.; Lee, K.; Park, S.K.; Kim, H.M.; Kwon, H.J.; Han, G. Property-based optimization of hydroxamate-based gamma-lactam HDAC inhibitors to improve their metabolic stability and pharmacokinetic profiles. *J. Med. Chem.,* 2012, *55*, 10766-10770.

[32] Zhang, Y.; Liu, H.; Jiao, Y.; Yuan, H.; Wang, F.; Lu, S.; Yao, S.; Ke, Z.; Tai, W.; Jiang, Y.; Chen, Y.; Lu, T. De novo design of N-(pyridin-4-ylmethyl)aniline derivatives as KDR inhibitors: 3D-QSAR, molecular fragment replacement, protein-ligand interaction fingerprint, and ADMET prediction. *Mol. Divers.,* 2012, *16*, 787-802.

[33] Aleksic, M.; Bertosa, B.; Nhili, R.; Uzelac, L.; Jarak, I.; Depauw, S.; David-Cordonnier, M.H.; Kralj, M.; Tomic, S.; Karminski-Zamola, G. Novel substituted benzothiophene and thienothiophene carboxanilides and quinolones: synthesis, photochemical synthesis, DNA-binding properties, antitumor evaluation and 3D-derived QSAR analysis. *J. Med. Chem.,* 2012, *55*, 5044-5060.

[34] Speck-Planche, A.; Kleandrova, V.V.; Luan, F.; Cordeiro, M.N.D.S. Unified Multi-target Approach for the Rational in silico Design of Anti-bladder Cancer Agents. *Anticancer Agents Med. Chem.,* 2013, *13*, 791-800.

[35] Prado-Prado, F.J.; Gonzalez-Diaz, H.; Santana, L.; Uriarte, E. Unified QSAR approach to antimicrobials. Part 2: predicting activity against more than 90 different species in order to halt antibacterial resistance. *Bioorg. Med. Chem.,* 2007, *15*, 897-902.

[36] Prado-Prado, F.J.; Borges, F.; Uriarte, E.; Perez-Montoto, L.G.; Gonzalez-Diaz, H. Multi-target spectral moment: QSAR for antiviral drugs vs. different viral species. *Anal. Chim. Acta,* 2009, *651*, 159-164.

[37] Prado-Prado, F.J.; Garcia-Mera, X.; Gonzalez-Diaz, H. Multi-target spectral moment QSAR versus ANN for antiparasitic drugs against different parasite species. *Bioorg. Med. Chem.,* 2010, *18*, 2225-2231.

[38] Alonso, N.; Caamano, O.; Romero-Duran, F.J.; Luan, F.; Cordeiro, M.N.D.S.; Yanez, M.; Gonzalez-Diaz, H.; Garcia-Mera, X. Model for High-Throughput Screening of Multi-Target Drugs in Chemical Neurosciences; Synthesis, Assay and Theoretic Study of Rasagiline Carbamates. *ACS Chem. Neurosci.,* 2013, *4*, 1393-1403.

[39] Gonzalez-Diaz, H.; Herrera-Ibata, D.M.; Duardo-Sanchez, A.; Munteanu, C.R.; Orbegozo-Medina, R.A.; Pazos, A. ANN Multiscale

Model of Anti-HIV Drugs Activity vs AIDS Prevalence in the US at County Level Based on Information Indices of Molecular Graphs and Social Networks. *J. Chem. Inf. Model.,* 2014, *54*, 744-755.

[40] Gonzalez-Diaz, H.; Prado-Prado, F.J. Unified QSAR and network-based computational chemistry approach to antimicrobials, part 1: multispecies activity models for antifungals. *J. Comput. Chem.,* 2008, *29*, 656-667.

[41] Vina, D.; Uriarte, E.; Orallo, F.; Gonzalez-Diaz, H. Alignment-free prediction of a drug-target complex network based on parameters of drug connectivity and protein sequence of receptors. *Mol. Pharmaceutics,* 2009, *6*, 825-835.

[42] Tenorio-Borroto, E.; Garcia-Mera, X.; Penuelas-Rivas, C.G.; Vasquez-Chagoyan, J.C.; Prado-Prado, F.J.; Castanedo, N.; Gonzalez-Diaz, H. Entropy model for multiplex drug-target interaction endpoints of drug immunotoxicity. *Curr. Top. Med. Chem.,* 2013, *13*, 1636-1649.

[43] Speck-Planche, A.; Cordeiro, M.N. Simultaneous Virtual Prediction of Anti-Escherichia coli Activities and ADMET Profiles: A Chemoinformatic Complementary Approach for High-Throughput Screening. *ACS Comb. Sci.,* 2014, *16*, 78-84.

[44] Speck-Planche, A.; Kleandrova, V.V.; Cordeiro, M.N.D.S. Chemoinformatics for rational discovery of safe antibacterial drugs: Simultaneous predictions of biological activity against streptococci and toxicological profiles in laboratory animals. *Bioorg. Med. Chem.,* 2013, *21*, 2727–2732.

[45] Speck-Planche, A.; Kleandrova, V.V.; Cordeiro, M.N.D.S. New insights toward the discovery of antibacterial agents: Multi-tasking QSBER model for the simultaneous prediction of anti-tuberculosis activity and toxicological profiles of drugs. *Eur. J. Pharm. Sci.,* 2013, *48*, 812-818.

[46] Speck-Planche, A.; Cordeiro, M.N.D.S. Simultaneous modeling of antimycobacterial activities and ADMET profiles: a chemoinformatic approach to medicinal chemistry. *Curr. Top. Med. Chem.,* 2013, *13*, 1656-1665.

[47] Tenorio-Borroto, E.; Penuelas-Rivas, C.G.; Vasquez-Chagoyan, J.C.; Castanedo, N.; Prado-Prado, F.J.; Garcia-Mera, X.; Gonzalez-Diaz, H. Model for high-throughput screening of drug immunotoxicity - Study of the anti-microbial G1 over peritoneal macrophages using flow cytometry. *Eur. J. Med. Chem.,* 2014, *72*, 206-220.

[48] Luan, F.; Cordeiro, M.N.D.S.; Alonso, N.; Garcia-Mera, X.; Caamano, O.; Romero-Duran, F.J.; Yanez, M.; Gonzalez-Diaz, H. TOPS-MODE model of multiplexing neuroprotective effects of drugs and

experimental-theoretic study of new 1,3-rasagiline derivatives potentially useful in neurodegenerative diseases. *Bioorg. Med. Chem.,* 2013, *21*, 1870–1879.

[49] Tenorio-Borroto, E.; Penuelas Rivas, C.G.; Vasquez Chagoyan, J.C.; Castanedo, N.; Prado-Prado, F.J.; Garcia-Mera, X.; Gonzalez-Diaz, H. ANN multiplexing model of drugs effect on macrophages; theoretical and flow cytometry study on the cytotoxicity of the anti-microbial drug G1 in spleen. *Bioorg. Med. Chem.,* 2012, *20*, 6181-6194.

[50] Speck-Planche, A.; Cordeiro, M.N.D.S. Evolution of Graph Theory-Based QSAR Methods and their Applications to the Search for New Antibacterial Agents. *Curr. Top. Med. Chem.,* 2013, *13*, 3101-3117.

[51] Gaulton, A.; Bellis, L.J.; Bento, A.P.; Chambers, J.; Davies, M.; Hersey, A.; Light, Y.; McGlinchey, S.; Michalovich, D.; Al-Lazikani, B.; Overington, J.P. ChEMBL: a large-scale bioactivity database for drug discovery. *Nucleic Acids Res.,* 2012, *40*, D1100-1107.

[52] Estrada, E.; Gutiérrez, Y. *MODESLAB*, v1.5; Santiago de Compostela, 2002-2004.

[53] Estrada, E. Spectral moments of the edge adjacency matrix in molecular graphs. 1. Definition and applications for the prediction of physical properties of alkanes. *J. Chem. Inf. Comput. Sci.,* 1996, *36*, 844–849.

[54] Estrada, E. Spectral moments of the edge adjacency matrix in molecular graphs. 2. Molecules containing heteroatoms and QSAR applications. *J. Chem. Inf. Comput. Sci.,* 1997, *37*, 320–328.

[55] Estrada, E. Spectral moments of the edge adjacency matrix in molecular graphs. 3. Molecules containing cycles. *J. Chem. Inf. Comput. Sci.,* 1998, *38*, 23–27.

[56] Hill, T.; Lewicki, P. *STATISTICS Methods and Applications. A Comprehensive Reference for Science, Industry and Data Mining*, StatSoft: Tulsa, 2006.

[57] Statsoft-Team. *STATISTICA. Data analysis software system*, v6.0; Tulsa, 2001.

[58] Speck-Planche, A.; Kleandrova, V.V.; Luan, F.; Cordeiro, M.N.D.S. Rational drug design for anti-cancer chemotherapy: multi-target QSAR models for the in silico discovery of anti-colorectal cancer agents. *Bioorg. Med. Chem.,* 2012, *20*, 4848-4855.

[59] Hanczar, B.; Hua, J.; Sima, C.; Weinstein, J.; Bittner, M.; Dougherty, E.R. Small-sample precision of ROC-related estimates. *Bioinformatics,* 2010, *26*, 822-830.

[60] Speck-Planche, A.; Kleandrova, V.V.; Luan, F.; Cordeiro, M.N.D.S. Fragment-based QSAR model toward the selection of versatile anti-sarcoma leads. *Eur. J. Med. Chem.,* 2011, *46*, 5910-5916.

In: Bladder Cancer
Editor: Samantha Haggerty
ISBN: 978-1-63321-666-2

Chapter 5

LONG NON CODING MITOCHONDRIAL RNAS AS POTENTIAL TARGETS FOR DIAGNOSIS AND THERAPY OF BLADDER CANCER

Jaime Villegas[1,2*†], Alexis Rivas[1†], Rodolfo Ávila[1†], Vincenzo Borgna[1,3†], Lorena Lobos-Gonzales[1†], Verónica Burzio,[1,2†], Constanza López,[1†] Reynaldo Gomez[3,4‡], Eduardo Landerer[3#], Laura Velarde[4‡] and L. O. Burzio[1,2†]

[1] Andes Biotechnologies S.A., Fundación Ciencia & Vida
[2] Facultad de Ciencias Biológicas
[3] Facultad de Medicina, Universidad Andrés Bello
[4] Unidad de Urología, Hospital de Trabajador. Santiago, Chile

[*] Corresponding author: jvillegas@bioschile.cl; Av. Zañartu 1482 – Ñuñoa. Santiago, Chile.
[†] Av. Zañartu 1482 – Ñuñoa.
[‡] Ramón Carnicer 185 – Providencia.
[#] Av. Republica 217 – Santiago.

Abstract

Bladder cancer (BC) is a heterogeneous disease with 70% of patients presenting superficial tumours and 30% presenting muscle-invading disease with a high risk of death associated to metastasis. The diagnosis is carried out by urine cytology, whith high specificity but low sensitivity, and cystoscopy, an expensive and unpleasant procedure. Carcinoma *in situ* and other high grade non-muscle-invasive tumors are treated by intravesical administration of BCG or other chemotherapeutic agents, while the indication for muscle-invasive disease is radical cystectomy.

Human cells express a family of mitochondrial long non-coding RNAs (ncRNAs). One of these transcripts, the sense mitochondrial ncRNA or SncmtRNA, is expressed in normal proliferating cells and tumor cells but not in non-dividing cells. In addition, normal human proliferating cells express two antisense transcripts, ASncmtRNA-1 and ASncmtRNA-2. Strikingly however, the ASncmtRNAs are down-regulated in tumor cell lines as well as in tumor cells present in different types of human cancer, including BC. Therefore, the differential expression profile of these transcripts allows to detect cancer cells in biopsies and biological fluids.

Down-regulation of the ASncmtRNAs seems to be an important hallmark of cancer and, hypothetically, may also represent a general vulnerability of cancer cells. Indeed, knock-down of the ASncmtRNAs using antisense oligonucleotides (ASO) exerts negative effects on cell proliferation and viability of bladder cancer cell lines representing a novel therapeutic strategy for this disease. We discuss recent advances on the use of the mitochondrial ncRNAs as targets for diagnostic and therapeutic protocols of BC and its potential use in the clinic.

Introduction

Among urological malignancies, bladder cancer (BC) is the most common, with an incidence four times higher in men than in women (Ploeg et al., 2009). BC comprises at least two major groups: low grade papillary tumors and high grade invasive tumors. Approximately 80% of BC are papillary and are treated by transurethral resections. They present, however, a high frequency of recurrence (up to 80% of cases) but rarely progress (McConkey et al., 2010). Unfortunately, patients with invasive disease have a much worse diagnosis, with only a 50% 5-year survival (Yang et al., 2004). The median ages of men and women diagnosed with BC are 72 and 74 years, respectively (Jemal et al., 2011), being old age the major risk factor of BC. Cigarrete smoking is another major risk factor, the relative risk of death from BC among smokers is 2, 75 times higher than in non-smokers (Brennan et al., 2000). Urinary tract infection, bladder stones, and a non-functioning bladder are associated with an increased risk of BC, specifically squamous cell carcinoma (SCC) (Shokeir, 2004).

Cystoscopy and urine cytology are the first line of clinical tools in the diagnosis and follow-up of bladder cancer. Cystoscopy an unpleasant and expensive procedure, is not always accurate when performed alone, and flat lesions (carcinoma *in situ*) and small papillary tumors can be missed (van Tilborg et al., 2009). In order to improve the diagnosis, new technologies have been developed, such as photodynamic diagnosis/blue-light (PDD) cystoscopy where 5-aminolevulinic acid is instilled into the bladder. Abnormal tissue is differentiated from normal, because these emits a red color under blue reference light (Cheung et al., 2013). The accuracy of urine cytology depends on several factors that are mainly related to tumor grade and sampling. Urine cytology is useful in the diagnosis of high-grade urothelial carcinoma. However, it carries a much lower diagnostic yield for papillary neoplasm of low malignant potential and low-grade papillary urothelial carcinoma, with sensitivity and specificity values as low as 8.5% and 50%, respectively (Raab et al., 2007). Therefore, cytology alone is too unreliable to serve as a decision-making criteria of therapeutic protocols.

In order to improve the widely noninvasive urine cytology, numerous urinary markers have been investigated. Several are commercially available, however no one has been adopted into clinical routine (Yutkin et al., 2010). ImmunoCyt/uCyt™ (DiagnoCure Inc., Québec, Canada) was aimed at improving the low sensitivity of cytology. This fluorescence test combines three monoclonal antibodies, raised against mucin-like antigen (Fradet et al., 1997). Several reports show that this test has low specificity and can be used mainly to postpone cystoscopies in patients followed for BC (Têtu et al., 2005; Greene et al., 2006). The BTA STAT and TRAK tests use monoclonal antibodies to detect complement factor H-related protein in voided urine. Sensitivity ranges between 58% and 72% and specificity between 48% and 75% (Messing et al., 2005). The NMP22 test uses a sandwich enzyme-linked immunosorbent assay with 2 monoclonal antibodies against the nuclear mitotic apparatus protein in urine and has a reported sensitivity between 47% and 81% and specificity between 64.3% and 93.3 (Hughes et al., 1999). These performance characteristics make it appealing when combined with cytology to help prolong the interval between cystoscopies in patients followed for bladder cancer.

Fluorescence *in situ* hybridization (FISH) is another noninvasive method for BC diagnosis. FISH is a rapid and powerful technique to detect cytogenetic abnormalities in malignant cells. For example, one commercial kit (UroVysion®; Abbot Molecular Inc.) uses fluorescently labeled probes to detect aneuploidy in chromosomes 3, 7 and 17, and loss of the 9p21 locus of the p16 tumor suppressor gene (Junker et al., 2003). The sensitivity of the UroVysion assay has been reported at 36% to 95%, and specificity, at 89% to 96% (Bubendorf et al., 2001). Despite its high performance across all stages and grades of bladder cancer there is a high false-positive rate and the test is very expensive and laborious (Halling, 2008).

Survivin, a member of the inhibitor of apoptosis gene family (Deveraux et al., 1999) is undetectable in most normal adult tissues, but is the top fourth transcript expressed in human cancers (Ambrosini et al,. 1997; Velculescu et al., 1999). Survivin was found in 78% of BC, but not in normal urothelium (Swana et al., 1999). Because of its differential expression pattern the potential suitability of urine survivin as new molecular marker has been investigated. Several studies show that determination of urine survivin transcript shows high sensitivity and specificity (Smith et al., 2001; Weikert et al., 2005). However, larger studies are needed to validate the diagnostic value of urinary survivin.

Transurethral resections of bladder tumor (TURBT) correspond to the first-line treatment for patients with non-muscle invasive bladder cancer; however, the high rate of recurrence after the procedure requires the use of adjuvant treatments. The most important therapeutic approaches are instillation of mitomycin-C, or immunotherapeutic agents such as Bacille Calmette-Guérin (BCG). They are the most adopted first-line immunotherapeutics and constitute the most effective treatment for prophylaxis and treatment of carcinoma *in situ* (CIS), either alone or in combination (Babjuk, et al., 2013). However, not all the patients can tolerate the side effects of hematuria or lower urinary-tract irritation, and are refractory to the treatment. In BCG-refractory patients other immunoregulators such as interferons (IFN), interleukin-2 (IL-2), interleukin-12 (IL-12), and tumor necrosis factor (TNF) have been used with varying results (Shen et al., 2008).

Besides mitomycin-C, multiple chemotherapeutic agents, such as doxorubicin, epirubicin, valrubicin, cisplatin, suramin or combinations of them have been evaluated in patients; meta-analyses did not show apparent superiority of any particular treatment (Ecke et al., 2006).

Recently, for metastatic BC, gemcitabine has been introduced, as chemotherapeutic agent (Shelley, et al., 2011). The methotrexate/vinblastine /doxorubicin/cisplatin combination is the standard treatment of this disease, with overall response rates of up to 72% and survival durations of approximately 1 year (Sternberg, 2000). With the addition of gemcitabine to the chemotherapeutic arsenal, approaches to bladder cancer are changing significantly. However, more studies are necessary to define the real efficacy of the drug, considering that some results obtained in clinical trials show only 28% of patients with a durable response (Skinner et al,. 2013).

Considering these features of BC, there is an urgent need to enhance anti-tumor effects of conventional treatments by specifically inactivating genes associated with obstacles to current therapies against BC. Of the current available strategies for gene silencing, antisense oligonucleotides (ASO) are the most widely used. ASO consist of short single-stranded DNA tipically 18 – 20 nucleotides in length and chemically modified to protect the ASO molecules against nucleases present in body fluids. One of these modifications is the introduction of phosphorothioate in the internucleosidic linkages where the phosphoryl oxygen is substituted for sulfur (ASO-PS); (McKay et al., 1999). Other modifications include 2'-O-methyl or 2'-O-methoxyethyl (2'MOE) substituents at the ribose (Gleave and Monia, 2005), locked nucleic acids (LNA) (Petersen and Wengel., 2003) and peptide nucleic acids (PNA), which belong to the third generation of ASOs (Petraccone et al., 2005).

A number of preclinical experiments evaluating the efficacies of ASO therapy for BC include targeting of antiapoptotic genes (bcl-2, survivin, clusterin, and hsp27), angiogenic factors (VEGF, IL-8 and bFGF), oncogenes (Hras and c-myc), growth factors (TGF-β1) and telomerase (Miyake et al., 2005; Fuessel et al., 2007; Miyake and Fujisawa, 2008).

Knockdown of the selected targets causes an impairment of growth of different BC cell lines, originating from cell cycle arrest or increased apoptosis. Moreover, pretreatment with ASO provoked strong enhancement of subsequent chemotherapy (Miyake et al., 2005). Therefore, ASO alone or in combination with chemotherapeutics agents might represent an alternative strategy for the treatment of BC.

Long Non-Coding RNAs in Bladder Cancer

Long non-coding RNAs (lncRNA) are non-protein coding transcripts longer than 200 nucleotides and, according to their genomic locations relative to protein coding genes, are classified in five broad categories: (1) sense or (2) antisense, (3) bidirectional, (4) intronic, and (5) intergenic (Gibb et al., 2011). The repertoire of lncRNA functions is rapidly expanding with defined roles in development and in several cell and molecular aspects of cell physiology, including mediators of mRNA decay (Gong and Maquat, 2011), host genes for miRNAs (Eis et al., 2005; Mestdagh et al., 2010), regulators of chromatin remodeling (Gupta et al., 2010) and scaffolds for nuclear substructures (Clemson et al., 2009). Beyond it multiple roles, accumulating evidence indicates aberrant expression of lncRNAs may play an important role in cancer biology (Gibb et al., 2011; Gutschner and Diederichs., 2012).

H19, the oldest known lncRNA is a paternally imprinted, maternally expressed transcript in human embryos and almost completely shut off in adults (Elkin et al., 1995). Nevertheless, H19 is re-expressed in several tumors, including bladder carcinoma. Ectopic expression of H19 promotes bladder cancer cell proliferation *in vitro* and enhances migration both *in vitro* and *in vivo* (Zho et al., 2012; Luo et al., 2013). Recently, a novel lncRNA, *linc*-UBC1 (Up-regulated in Bladder Cancer 1) was found to be over expressed in ~ 60% of invasive BCs and correlated with lymph node metastasis and low survival (Prensner et al., 2011). MALAT1 (Metastasis Associated Lung Adenocarcinoma Transcript 1) is up-regulated in BC and its expression is correlated with tumor grade and metastatic stage (Yin et al., 2012). In urothelial carcinoma, overexpression of MALAT1 induces cell proliferation, migration, and survival and activates the WNT pathway, promoting epithelial mesenchymal transition (EMT) required for migration, invasion and metastasis (Yin et al., 2012).

Maternally Expressed Gene 3 (MEG3) is expressed in many normal tissues, but its expression is lost in BC through multiple mechanisms, including gene deletion, promoter hypermethylation among others (Zhang et al., 2010). Down regulation of MEG3 in BC cells cause autophagy activation and increased cell proliferation (Zhou et al., 2012).

Expression of TUG1, Taurine up regulated gene 1, is associated with high grade and high stage BC and silencing of TUG1 in bladder cancer cells causes induction of apoptosis and inhibition of proliferation, supporting the oncogenic role of this lncRNA (Han et al., 2013). Another lncRNA with a role in BC is urothelial cancer associated 1 (UCA1), which is highly expressed in embryonic tissues and BC, but not in adult tissues or adjacent non-neoplastic tissues. Moreover, ectopic expression of UCA1 induces proliferation, migration, invasion and drug resistance, antagonizing cisplatin-induced apoptosis and promotes tumorogenicity *in vivo* (Wang et al., 2012; Yang et al., 2012; Tsang et al., 2007).

Regulatory Networks and lncRNAs in Bladder Cancer

The most prominent pathways responsible for promoting cell growth in BC are Ras-MAPK and PI3K-AKT-mTOR (Wu, 2005). Therefore an obvious question is whether lncRNAs are involved in regulation/dysregulation of these or other regulatory pathways. Very interesting relationships have been found between lncRNAs and regulatory circuits that play important roles in bladder cancer development and progression. For example, knock down of UCA1 in BLZ-211 cells causes a reduction in several cell cycle-related genes (CDKN2B, EP300 and TGFβ-2). Furthermore, activation of CREB and AKT are positively correlated with the level of UCA1 (Yang et al., 2012).

Activation of Wnt/β-catenin and subsequent down-regulation of E-cadherin results in over expression of H19 lncRNA, inducing loss of cellular adhesion and promotion of epithelial-mesenchymal transition, (EMT) (Lou et al., 2013). Moreover, hypoxia-induced H19 in bladder carcinoma increases the levels of genes involved in angiogenesis, cell survival, and proliferation (Ayesh et al., 2002; Matouk et al., 2007). Silencing of MALAT1 results in an increase of E-cadherin levels and decrease of the EMT-associated ZEB1, ZEB2 and Slug (Ying et al., 2012). Therefore, a core pathway targeted by lncRNAs seems to be Wnt signaling leading to tumorigenesis. Finally, autophagy contributes to survival of cancer cells; aberrant MEG3 expression in BC presents a negative correlation between autophagy levels LC3-II and MEG3 levels. Overexpression of this lncRNA markedly suppressed autophagy and increased apoptosis, whereas its knock-down activated autophagy and increased cell proliferation in bladder cancer cell lines (Zhang et al., 2003). Therefore, there is a strong association between the aberrant expression of MEG3 and autophagy and increase in cell proliferation in BC. Taken together, dysregulation of specific lncRNAs expression may represent potential novel biomarkers and might provide new therapeutic targets for the treatment of urological malignancies.

Mitochondrial lncRNAs in Bladder Cancer: Novel Tool for Diagnosis and Therapy

Human cells express a family of mitochondrial long non-coding RNAs (ncmtRNAs), containing steem-loop structures (Villegas et al., 2007, Burzio *et al*., 2009). A functional role of these molecules outside the mitochondria is suggested by the cytoplasmic and nuclear localization of these transcripts determined by electron microscopy *in situ* hybridization (Landerer et al., 2011). One of these transcripts, sense ncmtRNA (SncmtRNA) is expressed in normal proliferating cells, as well as in tumor cells but not in non-dividing cells, suggesting a role in cell cycle progression. This correlation of SncmtRNA with the proliferative status of cells is supported by several experimental data. Treatment of HeLa cells with ethidium bromide, which specifically inhibits mtDNA replication and transcription, blocks cell proliferation and expression of the SncmtRNA (Villegas et al., 2007). In addition, rhodamine 6G, a drug that disables mitochondrial function (Felty et al., 2005) inhibits, in a reversible manner the expression of the SncmtRNA, together with DNA synthesis and PCNA expression in phytohemagglutinin-stimulated human lymphocytes (Burzio et al., 2009). After removal of the drug, DNA synthesis and PCNA and SncmtRNA expression are reestablished. On the other hand, knock-down of the SncmtRNA in HeLa and SiHa cells (transformed with HPV 18 or 16, respectively) induces strong inhibition of cell proliferation (Villota et al., 2012). Normal proliferating cells also express two antisense transcripts named ASncmtRNA-1 and -2. Remarkably however, tumor cells lines, as well as tumor cells present in seventeen types of human cancer, down-regulate the expression of ASncmtRNAs (Burzio et al., 2009). A characteristic or hallmark of carcinogenesis is down-regulation of tumor suppressors involving several mechanisms (Payne and Kemp, 2005). We hypothesized that, because the ASncmtRNAs were down regulated in tumor cell lines and biopsies of different types of cancer, these transcripts constitute tumor suppressors, like other non-coding RNAs (miRs and LncRNAs). Therefore, the ASncmtRNAs might function as unique mitochondria-encoded tumor suppressors. To test this possibility, we used normal human keratinocytes immortalized with high risk human papillomaviruses (HPV) 16 and 18. Immortalization of normal keratinocytes by these viruses is mediated by the viral oncoproteins E6 and E7 which abolish the function of the tumor suppressors Rb and p53 (Payne and Kemp, 2005). In keratinocytes immortalized with the complete genome of HPV 16 or 18 the ASncmtRNAs are also down regulated (Villota et al., 2012). Therefore, we hypothesize that an oncogene(s) of HPV16 or HPV 18 could be involved in down regulation of the ASncmtRNAs. Indeed we found that the E2 protein of these viruses was responsible of down regulation of these transcripts (Villota et al., 2012). These results support our hypothesis that the ASncmtRNAs are tumor suppressors, and we theorize that in non-viral-induced cancers, down-regulation of the

ASncmtRNAs could be triggered by as yet undetermined cellular oncogenes (Villota et al., 2012). Therefore, down-regulation of the ASncmtRNAs seems to be an important step in carcinogenesis and represents a new and generalized hallmark of cancer in addition to those defined by Hannahan and Weinberg (2011).

The remarkable differential expression of the SncmtRNA and the ASncmtRNAs distinguishes normal proliferating cells from malignant cells as illustrated in Figure 1 (Burzio et al., 2009). FISH shows that the BC cell line T24 expresses the SncmtRNA (green) but not the ASncmtRNAs (red). In contrast, normal proliferating renal epithelial cells express both types of transcripts. Recently, and based on this differential expression pattern, we performed a pilot study in biopsies of cervical cancer, showing that down-regulation of ASncmtRNAs is found as early as cervical intraepithelial neoplasia, grade I (CIN I) and, support the possibility of using this differential expression as a diagnostic tool for cervical cancer (Villegas et al,. 2013)

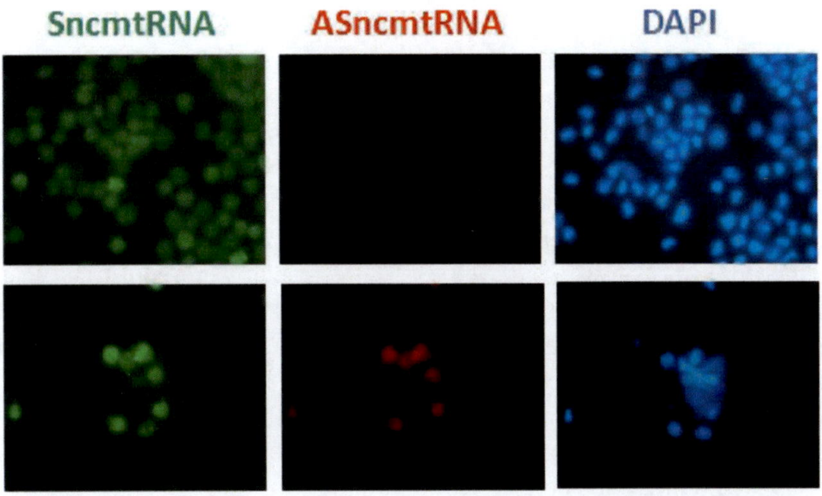

Figure 1. Differential expression of ncmtRNAs in normal proliferating cells and tumor cells. Bladder cancer cells (T24, upper) and normal proliferating cells, corresponding to renal cells (down), were hybridized simultaneously with probes against the SncmtRNA (green labeled probe, Alexa Fluor 488) and ASncmtRNA (Red-labeled probe, Texas Red). Normal proliferating cells express both RNAs at the same level and, tumor cells down-regulate only the ASncmtRNA. To visualize all the cells, DAPI was used to indicate the presence of cells. This expression pattern distinguishes tumor cells from normal cells.

A preliminary pilot study in our laboratory showed that in bladder cancer biopsies corresponding to different stages (grade I, II, and III), only the SncmtRNA is detected (Figure 2). Depending of the stage, the staining pattern is principally nuclear (grade III) or cytoplasmic (grade II) and, in the case of grade I, a nuclear/cytoplasmic distribution of the staining is observed. However, at present we do not know if there is any relationship between the signal pattern of the ncmtRNAs and prognosis of disease progression, and this matter is presently under study.

Since down-regulation of the ASncmtRNAs seems to be independent of BC stage, the differential expression pattern of these transcripts (see Figure 1) can be applied as a diagnostic method. Therefore, we developed a non-invasive and single protocol to detect the expression of these molecules in the urine of patients with BC. Because voided urine is an important source of exfoliated cells, cytological examination of the sediment of voided urine is the only noninvasive method of detection, diagnosis and follow-up of tumors of the bladder and other anatomic components of the lower urinary tract (Koss et al., 1985).

Fluorescence *in situ* hybridization (FISH) is a powerful technique that can detect chromosomal abnormalities that are associated with several malignancies, including BC. The use of FISH in conjunction with urine cytology can potentially reduce urothelial carcinoma morbidity and mortality at the earliest stage of these tumors. Sokolova et al reported a FISH assay with high sensitivity and specificity for high grade BC. The protocol include four labeled probes specific to chromosomes 3, 7, and 17 and a locus-specific probe to band 9p21 (Sokolova *et al.*, 2000). These results were confirmed in later studies with a large cohort of patients (Kang et al., 2006; Kipp et al., 2009). These studies support this promising application of FISH and was latter approved by the FDA as a commercial kit, Urovysion® (Abbot Molecular/Vysis, Des Plaines, IL). However, multiple studies shown that this test has low sensitivity, for low-stage and low-grade tumors (Bubendorf and Piaton, 2012; Dimaskieh et al., 2013).

We developed a one-tube FISH protocol applied to cells in suspension (S-FISH), that takes about 60 minutes to perform and uses simultaneously, two fluorescently labeled probes for SncmtRNA (green-labeled probe) and ASncmtRNA (red-labeled probe), method that was applied to cells isolated from voided urine of patients with BC (Rivas et al., 2012).

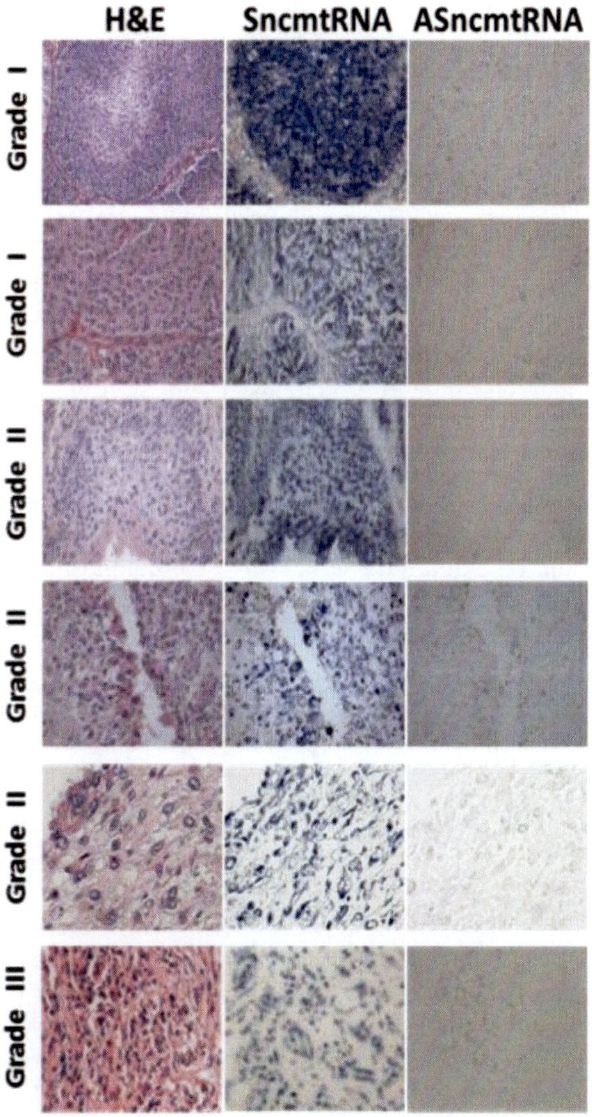

Figure 2. Expression of SncmtRNA and ASncmtRNAs in bladder cancer biopsies of different malignant grades. Parallel biopsy sections corresponding to BC of different stages were subjected to ISH for S- and ASncmtRNAs. Down-regulation of the AS transcript is observed in all cases (ASncmtRNA). A parallel section was stained with Hematoxylin & Eosin (H&E). (x 400).

For the FISH protocol we developed, cells were collected by centrifugation from cell culture or from biological fluids such as urine and blood, followed by permeabilization with 0.2 N HCl. After neutralization, the cells were recovered, hybridized with probes for the SncmtRNA (labeled with Alexas fluor 488) and for the ASncmtRNAs (conjugated to Texas Red), washed and analyzed by fluorescence microscopy. The test is reproducible and has been applied to tumor cell lines and normal cells. Hybridization of normal proliferating cells added to voided urine (human umbilical vein endothelial cells, keratinocytes and melanocytes) readily detects the SncmtRNA and the ASncmtRNAs. In addition, the hybridization signal was not affected by incubation of cells in urine for 24 to 48 h.

Our pilot study was able to detect cancer cells in urine from twenty-four patients with BC and the results were independent of the grade of BC and cellularity. In the case of healthy donors, cells were recovered only from six out of fifteen samples and the S-FISH showed absence of signal to both transcripts (Rivas et al., 2012). Therefore, these preliminary results suggest that S-FISH could be explored as a non-invasive diagnostic tool for bladder cancer. At present we are evaluating in a double-blind protocol, a cohort of 180 patients that include healthy individuals, BC, non-infectious acute inflammation and infectious acute inflammation of the urinary track.

As mentioned before, down-regulation of ASncmtRNAs could play an important role in carcinogenesis, representing a new and generalized hallmark of cancer (Hanahan and Weinberg, 2011, Vidaurre et al., 2014). Therefore, we hypothesized that down-regulation of the AS transcript may also represent a general vulnerability of cancer cells. In order to explore this hypothesis we performed knockdown of the ASncmtRNAs using antisense oligonucleotides (ASO-PS) in several tumor cell lines. Treatment of cells with 100nM ASO-PS for 48h shows a strong inhibition of proliferation rate, induction of caspase activation and other hallmarks of apoptosis (Vidaurre et al., 2014). Moreover, ASO treatment induces a drastic reduction in the levels of survivin, a member of the inhibitor of apoptosis (IAP) family, which is up regulated in practically all human cancers (Altieri, 2010; Kang et al., 2011).

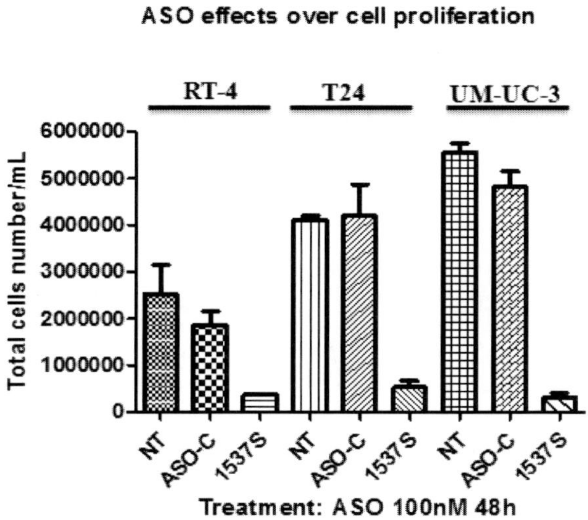

a

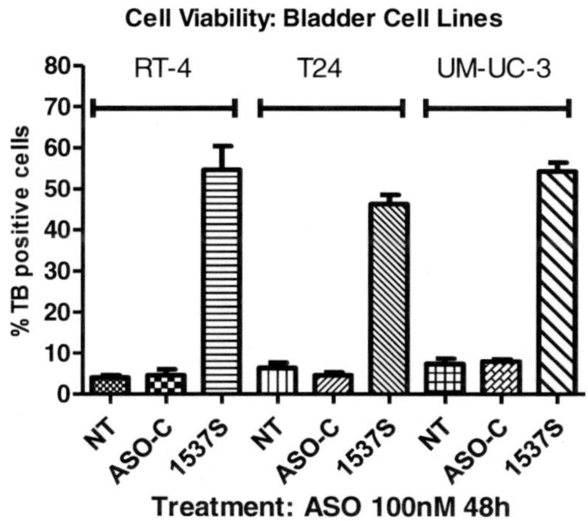

b

Figure 3. Effects on cell proliferation and cell viability after antisense treatment in three different cell lines of bladder cancer. In a 12-well plate, 50.000 cells of each cell line were seeded, transfected with the ASOs indicated and, after 48h, cells were trypsinized and the efficacy of treatment was determined by trypan blue (TB) exclusion assay. A) Total cell numbers after treatment, B) Trypan blue assay. Non treated cells (NT), as wells as treated with control ASO (ASO-C), show a basal death level. Cells treated with ASO against the ASncmtRNAs (ASO 1537S), display an average cell death of 50% in three cell lines. Each experiment was performed in triplicate.

An important point is that the same treatments that induce massive cell death in tumor cells do not affect the viability of normal proliferating cells. The resistance mechanism of normal cells is unclear but a possible explanation is that survivin is practically undetectable in normal cells and, in contrast to cancer cells, is not localized in the mitochondria (Dohi et al, 2007). Taken together, these results suggest that the ASncmtRNAs are promising targets for cancer therapy (Vidaurre et al., 2014).

Therefore, we asked whether ASncmtRNA knockdown (ASK) induces cell death in bladder tumor cell lines. In this context, we examined the effects of ASO-PS against the ASncmtRNAs on three-cell lines representative of the disease and encompassing different malignancy grades and genetic content. RT-4 (wild-type p53, CDKN2A mutant), T24 (HRAS and p53 mutants) and UM-UC-3 (p53, KRAS and PTEN mutated).

We found that, independent of the malignancy grade of BC cell lines, ASK induces a strong inhibition of cell proliferation and massive cell death evaluated by trypan blue exclusion assay in three BC cell lines (Figure 3). The cell death average after 48h of treatment is around 55% (see 1537S in Figure 3). However, cells treated with control oligonucleotide (ASO-C) show the same levels of death induction as non-treated cells (NT). Moreover, experimental evidence show that ASK induces DNA fragmentation (assessed by TUNEL assay), a drastic reduction in the migratory and invasive properties of the tumor cell lines *in vitro*, and reduction in tumorigenic properties (colony formation), stemness (sphere formation) and metastasis (Lobos-Gonzales et al., 2014, in preparation).

These results indicate that ASncmtRNAs are potential therapeutic targets for BC. We are performing protocols to assess the efficacy of ASK *in vivo* in murine models using at least two experimental approaches: sub-cutaneous injection of BC cells in xenograft experiments and syngeneic orthotropic models in order to evaluate the efficacy of ASK *in vivo* under different ASO injection regimes.

PERSPECTIVES

Dysregulation of ncmtRNAs in bladder cancer could constitute novel targets for both diagnosis, prognosis and treatment of cancer. Mitochondrial non-coding RNAs are relative stable in cells present in urine sample and the differential expression of ncmtRNAs (sense and antisense) in cells isolated of voided urine of patients with BC was used as proof-of-concept of a noninvasive diagnostic assay (Rivas et al., 2012). However, in order to validate this protocol as a diagnostic method it is necessary to carry out a study using a large cohort of patients with several related urological diseases, study that is presently in process.

For bladder cancer, the goal of administration of ASO is local tumor control, including both inhibition of recurrence and, ideally, precluding progression to muscle-invasive tumours. The bladder represents a "perfect" organ, i.e, the drug or ASO can be delivered *in situ*, without "dilution" in the blood stream, the relative low number of cellular layers represents an easy barrier for penetration of the therapeutic agents into deep tissue layers and *in situ* administration of ASO represents a minimal systemic toxic risk.

Down-regulation of ASncmtRNAs observed in tumor cells represents a novel therapeutic target which, upon specific interference by ASO-PS induces massive cell death, mediated by apoptosis and down-regulation of survivin. The usefulness of this promising ASO-based therapy must be proven in preclinical assays, used alone or as neo-adjuvant therapy in order to translate to clinical assays.

FUNDING: INNOVA-CORFO 12IDL4-13358 and 12IEAT-16317, CCTE-PFB16 Program, Conicyt, Chile.

REFERENCES

Altieri, D.C. (2010). Survivin and IAP proteins in cell-death mechanisms. *Biochem J,* 430, 199-205.

Ambrosini, G. Adida, C. & Altieri, D. (1997). A novel anti-apoptosis gene, survivin, expressed in cancer and lymphoma. *Nature Medicine* 3, 917–921.

Angela, A.G; Van Tilborg, Chris H Bangma and Ellen C Zwarthoff. (2009). Bladder cancer biomarkers and their role in surveillance and screening. *International Journal of Urology,* 16, 23–30.

Ayesh, S. Matouk, I. Schneider, T. Ohana, P. Laster, M. Al-Sharef, W. De-Groot, N. & Hochberg, A. (2002). Possible physiological role of H19 RNA. *Mol Carcinog,* 35, 63-74.

Babjuk, M. Burger, M. Zigeuner, R. Shariat, S. Bas, W.G. van Rhijn. Comperat, E. Sylvester, R. Kaasinen, E. Bohle, A. Redorta, J.P. & Roupret, M. (2013). EAU Guidelines on Non–Muscle-invasive Urothelial Carcinoma of the Bladder: Update 2013. European Urology, 64, 639–653.

Brennan, P. Bogillot, O. Cordier, S. Greiser, E. Schill, W. Vineis, P. Lopez-Abente, G. Tzonou, A. Chang-Claude, J. Bolm-Audorff, U. Jöckel, K. Donato, F. Serra, C. Wahrendorf, J. Hours, M. T'Mannetje, A. Kogevinas, M. & Boffetta, P. (2000). Cigarette smoking and bladder cancer in men: A pooled analysis of 11 case-control studies. *International Journal of Cancer,* 86, 289–294.

Bubendorf, L. Grilli, B. Sauter, G. et al. (2001). Multiprobe FISH for enhanced detection of bladder cancer in voided urine specimens and bladder washings. *Am J Clin Pathol,* 116, 79–86.

Bubendorf, L. Grilli, B. Sauter, G. Mihatsch, M. Gasser, T. & Dalquen P. (2001). Multiprobe FISH for Enhanced Detection of Bladder Cancer in Voided Urine Specimens and Bladder Washings. *Am J Clin Pathol,* 116, 79-86.

Bubendorf, L. & Piaton, E. (2012). UroVysion® multiprobe FISH in the triage of equivocal urinary cytology cases. *Ann Pathol,* 32, 438-43.

Burzio, V.A. Villota, C. Villegas, J. Landerer, E. Boccardo, E. Villa, L, L. Martínez, R. Lopez, C. Gaete, F. Toro, V. Rodriguez, X. & Burzio, L. O. (2009). Expression of a family of noncoding mitochondrial RNAs distinguishes normal from cancer cells. *Proc Natl Acad Sci U S A,* 106, 9430-9434.

Clemson, C.M. Hutchinson, J. N. Sara, S.A. Ensminger, A. W. Fox, A.H. Chess, A. & Lawrence, J.B. (2009). An architectural role for a nuclear noncoding RNA: NEAT1 RNA is essential for the structure of paraspeckles. *Mol Cell,* 27,717-726.

Cheung, G. Sahai, A. Billia, M. Dasgupta, P. & Khan, M.S. (2013). Recent advances in the diagnosis and treatment of bladder cancer. *BMC Medicine,* 11, 13.

David, J. McConkey, Sangkyou, Lee. Woonyoung, Choi. Mai, Tran. Tadeusz, Majewski, Sooyong Lee, Arlene Siefker-Radtke, Colin Dinney, & Bogdan, C. (2010). Molecular genetics of bladder cancer: Emerging mechanisms of tumor initiation and progression. *Urol Oncol,* 28, 429–440.

Deveraux, Q. & Reed, J.C. (1999). IAP family proteins—suppressors of apoptosis. *Genes & Development,* 13,239–252.

Dimashkieh, H. Wolff, D.J. Smith, T.M. Houser, P.M. Nietert, P.J. & Yang. (2013) Evaluation of urovysion and cytology for bladder cancer detection: a study of 1835 paired urine samples with clinical and histologic correlation. *J. Cancer Cytopathol,* 121,591-597.

Dohi, T. Xia, F. & Altieri, D. (2007). Compartmentalized phosphorylation of IAP by protein kinase A regulates cytoprotection. *Mol Cell,* 27, 17–28.

Ecke, T. Bartel, P. Koch, S. Ruttloff, J. & Theissig, F. (2006). Chemotherapy with gemcitabine, paclitaxel, and cisplatin in the treatment of patients with advanced transitional cell carcinoma of the urothelium. *Oncol. Rep,* 16, 1381–1388.

Eis, P.S. Tam, W. Sun, L. Chadburn, A. Li, Z. Gomez, M,F. Lund, E. & Dahlberg, J.E. (2005). Accumulation of miR-155 and BIC RNA in human B cell lymphomas. *Proc Natl Acad Sci U S A,* 8, 102(10):

Elkin, M. Shevelev, A. Schulze, E. Tykocinsky, M. Cooper, M. Ariel, I. Pode, D. Kopf, E. de Groot, N. & Hochberg, A. (1995). The expression of the imprinted H19 and IGF-2 genes in human bladder carcinoma. *FEBS Lett,* 23, 57-61.

Felty, Q. Singh, K.P. & Roy, D. (2005). Estrogen-induced G1/S transition of G0-arrested estrogen-dependent breast cancer cells is regulated by mitochondrial oxidant signaling. *Oncogene,* 24, 4883-4893.

Fradet, Y. & Lockhard, C. (1997). Performance characteristics of a new monoclonal antibody test for bladder cancer: ImmunoCyt trade mark. *Can J Urol,* 4, 400–405.

Fuessel, S. Meye, A. Kraemer, K. Kunze, D. Hakenberg, O. & Wirth, M. (2007). Synthetic nucleic acids as potential therapeutic tools for treatment of bladder carcinoma. *Eur Urol,* 51,315-326.

Gibb, E.A. Vucic, E.A. Enfield, K.S. Stewart, G.L. Lonergan, K.M. Kennett, J.Y. Becker-Santos, D.D. MacAulay, C.E. Lam, S. Brown, C.J. & Lam, W.L. (2011). Human cancer long non-coding RNA transcriptomes. *PLoS One,* 6, e25915.

Gleave, M.E. & Monia, B.P. (2005). Antisense therapy for cancer. Nat Rev Cancer, 6,468-479.

Gong, C. & Maquat, L.E. (2011). lncRNAs transactivate STAU1-mediated mRNA decay by duplexing with 3' UTRs via Alu elements. *Nature,* 10, 284-288.

Grace, C. Arun, S. Michele, B. Prokar, D. & Muhammad, S. (2013). Recent advances in the diagnosis and treatment of bladder cancer. *BMC Medicine,* 11:13.

Greene, K. Berry, A. & Konety, B. (2006). Diagnostic Utility of the ImmunoCyt/uCyt+ Test in Bladder Cancer. *Rev Urol*, 8, 190–197.

Grossman, S. Anthony, J.N. Weiss, R.M. & Altieri, D.C. (1999). Tumor content of the antiapoptosis molecule survivin and recurrence of bladder cancer. *N Engl J Med,* 341,452–453.

Gupta, R.A. Shah, N. Wang, K.C. Kim, J. Horlings, H.M. Wong, D.J. Tsai, M.C. Hung, T. Argani, P. Rinn, J.L. Wang, Y. Brzoska, P. Kong, B. Li, R. West, R.B. van de Vijver, M.J. Sukumar, S. & Chang, H.Y. (2010). Long non-coding RNA HOTAIR reprograms chromatin state to promote cancer metastasis. *Nature,* 464, 1071-1076.

Gutschner, T. & Diederichs, S. (2012). The hallmarks of cancer: a long non-coding RNA point of view. *RNA Biol,* 6,703-719.

Halling, K. & Kipp, B. (2008). Bladder Cancer Detection Using FISH (UroVysion Assay). *Adv Anat Pathol,* 15, 279–286.

Han, Y. Liu, Y. Gui, Y. & Cai, Z. (2013). Long intergenic non-coding RNA TUG1 is overexpressed in urothelial carcinoma of the bladder. *J Surg Oncol,* 107, 555-559.

Hanahan, D. & Weinberg, R.A. (2011). Hallmarks of cancer: the next generation. *Cell,* 144, 646-674.

Hughes, J.H. Katz, R.L. Rodriguez-Villanueva, J. Kidd, L. Dinney, C. Grossman, H.B. & Fritsche, H.A Jr. (1999) Urinary nuclear matrix protein 22 (NMP22): a diagnostic adjunct to urine cytologic examination for the detection of recurrent transitional-cell carcinoma of the bladder. *Diagn Cytopathol,* 20, 285–290.

Jemal, A. Bray, F. Center, M. Ferlay, J. Ward, E. & Forman, D. (2011). Global cancer statistics. CA: *A Cancer Journal for Clinicians,* 61, 69–90.

Junker, K. Boernera, D. Schulzeb, W. Uttinga, M. Schuberta, J. & Wernera. W. (2003). Analysis of genetic alterations in normal bladder urothelium. *Urology* 62, 1134–1138.

Kang, J.U. Koo, S.H. Jeong, T.E. Kwon, K.C. Park, J.W. & Jeon, C.H. (2006). Multitarget fluorescence in situ hybridization and melanoma antigen genes analysis in primary bladder carcinoma. *Cancer Genet Cytogenet*, 164, 32-38.

Kang, Y.J. Kim, I.Y. Kim, E.H. Yoon, M.J. Kim, S.U. Kwon, T.K. & Choi, K.S. (2011). Paxilline enhances TRAIL-mediated apoptosis of glioma cells via modulation of c-FLIP, survivin and DR5. *Exp Mol Med,* 43, 24–34.

Kipp, B.R. Tanasescu, M. Else, T.A. Bryant, S.C. Karnes, R.J. Sebo, T.J. & Halling, K.C. (2009). Quantitative fluorescence in situ hybridization and its ability to predict bladder cancer recurrence and progression to muscle-invasive bladder cancer. *J Mol Diagn,* 11, 148-154.

Koss, L.G. Deitch, D. Ramanathan, R. Sherman, A.B. (1985). Diagnostic value of cytology of voided urine. *Acta Cytol*, 5, 810-816.

Landerer, E. Villegas, J. Burzio, V.A. Oliveira, L. Villota, C. Lopez, C. Restovic, F. Martinez, R. Castillo, O. & Burzio, L.O. (2011). Nuclear localization of the mitochondrial ncRNAs in normal and cancer cells. *Cell Oncol,* 34, 97-305.

Lobos, L. Borgna, V. Ávila, R. Silva, V. Rivas, A. López, C. Socias, T. Landerer, E. Burzio, L.O. & Villegas, J. (2014). Targeted inhibition of antisense non coding mitochondrial RNA promotes apoptosis, inhibits invasion and tumorigenic properties in human urinary bladder cancer cell lines. (in preparation).

Luo, M. Li, Z. Wang, W. Zeng, Y. Liu, Z. Qiu, J. (2013). Long non-coding RNA H19 increases bladder cancer metastasis by associating with EZH2 and inhibiting E-cadherin expression. *Cancer Lett,* 10,213-221.

Matouk, I.J. DeGroot, N. Mezan, S. Ayesh, S. Abu-lail, R. Hochberg, A. & Galun, E. (2007). The H19 non-coding RNA is essential for human tumor growth. *PLoS One,* 2, e845.

McKay, R.A. Miraglia, L.J. Cummins, L,L. Owens, S.R. Sasmor, H. & Dean, N.M. (1999). Characterization of a potent and specific class of antisense oligonucleotide inhibitor of human protein kinase C-alpha expression. *J Biol Chem.* 274, 1715-1722.

Messing, E.M. Teot, L. Korman, H. Underhill, E. Barker, E. Stork, B. Qian, J. & Bostwick, D.G. (2005). Performance of urine test in patients monitored for recurrence of bladder cancer: a multicenter study in the United States. *J Urol,* 174, 1238–1241.

Mestdagh, P. Boström, A.K. Impens, F. Fredlund, E. Van Peer, G. De Antonellis, P. von Stedingk, K. Ghesquière, B. Schulte, S. Dews, M. Thomas-Tikhonenko, A. Schulte, J.H. Zollo, M. Schramm, A. Gevaert, K. Axelson, H. Speleman, F. & Vandesompele, J. (2010). The miR-17-92 microRNA cluster regulates multiple components of the TGF-β pathway in neuroblastoma. *Mol Cell,* 40,762-773.

Miyake, H. & Fujisawa, M. (2008). Promise of antisense oligodeoxynucleotide-based therapy for bladder cancer. *Expert Rev Anticancer Ther,* 8, 1851-1854.

Miyake, H. Hara, I. Fujisawa, M. & Gleave, M.E. (2005). Antisense oligodeoxynucleotide therapy for bladder cancer: recent advances and future prospects. *Expert Rev Anticancer Ther,* 6, 1001-1009.

Miyake, H. Yamanaka, K. Muramaki, M. Hara, I. & Gleave, M.E. (2005). Therapeutic efficacy of adenoviral-mediated p53 gene transfer is synergistically enhanced by combined use of antisense oligodeoxynucleotide targeting clusterin gene in a human bladder cancer model. *Neoplasia,* 7, 171-179.

Payne, S.R. and Kemp, C.J. (2005). Tumor suppressor genetics. *Carcinogenesis*, 26, 2031-2045.

Petersen, M. & Wengel, J. (2003). LNA: a versatile tool for therapeutics and genomics. *Trends Biotechnol,* 2, 74-81.

Petraccone, L. Pagano, B. Esposito, V. Randazzo, A. Piccialli, G. Barone, G. Mattia, C.A. & Giancola, C. (2005). Thermodynamics and kinetics of PNA-DNA quadruplex-forming chimeras. *J Am Chem Soc,* 127, 16215-16223.

Ploeg, M. Aben, K. & Kiemeney, L. (2009). The present and future burden of urinary bladder cancer in the world. *World J Urol,* 27, 289–293.

Prensner, J.R. & Chinnaiyan, A.M. (2011). The emergence of lncRNAs in cancer biology. *Cancer Discov,* 1, 391–407.

Raab, S. Grzybicki, D. Vrbin, C. & Geisinger, K. (2007). Urine Cytology Discrepancies Frequency, Causes, and Outcomes. *American Journal of Clinical Pathology,* 127, 946-953.

Raab, S.S. Grzybicki, D.M. Vrbin, C.M. & Geisinger, K. (2007). Urine cytology discrepancies: frequency, causes, and outcomes. *Am J Clin Pathol,* 127, 946–953.

Rivas, A. Burzio, V. Landerer, E. Borgna, V. Gatica, S. Ávila, R. López, C. Villota, C. de la Fuente, R. Echenique, J. Burzio, L.O. & Villegas, J. (2012). Determination of the differential expression of mitochondrial long non-coding RNAs as a noninvasive diagnosis of bladder cancer. *BMC Urol,* 18; 12:37.

Shelley, M. Cleves, A. Wilt, T. & Mason, M. (2011). Gemcitabine chemotherapy for the treatment of metastatic bladder carcinoma. *BJU International,* 108, 168–179.

Shen, Z. Shen, T. Wientjes, M. O'Donnell, M. & Jessie, L. (2008). Intravesical Treatments of Bladder Cancer *Pharm Res,* 25, 1500–1510.

Shokeir, A. (2004). Squamous cell carcinoma of the bladder: pathology, diagnosis and treatment. *BJU Int,* 93, 216–220.

Skinner, E.C. Goldman, B. Sakr, W.A. Petrylak, D.P. Lenz, H.J. Lee, C.T. Wilson, S.S. Benson, M. Lerner, S.P. Tangen, C.M. & Thompson, I.M. (2013). SWOG S0353: Phase II trial of intravesical gemcitabine in patients with nonmuscle invasive bladder cancer and recurrence after 2 prior courses of intravesical bacillus Calmette-Guérin. *J Urol,* 190, 1200-1204.

Smith, S. Wheeler, M. Plescia, J. Colberg, J. Weiss, R. & Altieri, D. (2001). Urine Detection of Survivin and Diagnosis of Bladder Cancer. *JAMA,* 285, 324-328.

Sokolova, I.A. Halling, K.C. Jenkins, R.B. Burkhardt, H.M. Meyer, R.G. Seelig, S.A. & King, W. (2000). The development of a multitarget, multicolor fluorescence in situ hybridization assay for the detection of urothelial carcinoma in urine. *J Mol Diagn,* 2,116-123.

Tetu, B. Tiguert, R. Harel, F. & Fradet, I. (2005) ImmunoCyt/uCyt+ improves the sensitivity of urine cytology in patients followed for urothelial carcinoma. *Mod Pathol,* 18, 83–89.

Tsang, W.P. Wong, T.W. Cheung, A.H. Co, C.N. & Kwok, T.T. (2007). Induction of drug resistance and transformation in human cancer cells by the noncoding *RNA CUDR. RNA,* 13, 890–898.

Van Tilborg, A. A. Bangma, C. H. & Zwarthoff, E. C. (2009). Bladder cancer biomarkers and their role in surveillance and screening. *International Journal of Urology,* 16, 23–30.

Velculescu, V. E. Madden, S. L. Zhang, L. Lash, A. E. Yu, J. Rago, C. Lal, A. Wang, C.J. Beaudry, G.A. Ciriello, K.M. et al. (1999). Analysis of human transcriptomes. *Nat. Genet,* 23, 387-388.

Vidaurre, S. Fitzpatrick, C. Burzio, V.A. Briones, M. Villota, C. Villegas, J. Echenique, J. Oliveira-Cruz, L. Araya, M. Borgna, V. Socías, T. Lopez, C. Avila, R. & Burzio, L.O. (2014). Down-regulation of the Antisense Mitochondrial ncRNAs is a Unique Vulnerability of Cancer Cells and a Potential Target for Cancer Therapy. *J. Biol. Chem.*

Villegas, J. Dadlani, K. Avila, R. Villota, C. Burzio, V. Lopez, C. Socias, M. Zapata, L. & Burzio, L.O. (2013). The Mitochondrial Antisense ncRNAs are Down-Regulated in Early Cervical Carcinoma. *J Cancer Sci Ther,* S7.

Villegas, J. Burzio, V. Villota, C. Landerer, E. Martinez, R. Santander, M. Pinto, R. Vera, M.I. Boccardo, E. Villa, L.L. & Burzio, L.O. (2007). Expression of a novel non-coding mitochondrial RNA in human proliferating cells. *Nucleic Acids Res,* 35, 7336-7347.

Villota, C. Campos, A. Vidaurre, S. Oliveira-Cruz, L. Boccardo, E. Burzio, V.A. Varas, M. Villegas, J. Villa, L.L. Valenzuela, P.D. Socías, M. Roberts, S. & Burzio, L.O. (2012). Expression of mitochondrial non-coding RNAs (ncRNAs) is modulated by high risk human papillomavirus (HPV) oncogenes. *J Biol Chem,* 287, 21303-21315.

Wang, Y. Chen, W. Yang, C. Wu, W. Wu, S. Qin, X. & Li, X. (2012). Long non-coding RNA UCA1a (CUDR) promotes proliferation and tumorigenesis of bladder cancer. *Int J Oncol,* 41, 276-284.

Weikert, S. Christoph, F. Schrader, M. Krause, H. Miller, K. & Müller, M. (2005). Quantitative analysis of survivin mRNA expression in urine and tumor tissue of bladder cancer patients and its potential relevance for disease detection and prognosis. *Int. J. Cancer,* 116, 100–104.

Wu, X.R. (2005). Urothelial tumorigenesis: a tale of divergent pathways. *Nat Rev Cancer,* 92, 80–88.

Yang, C. Li, X. Wang, Y. Zhao, L. & Chen, W. (2012). Long non-coding RNA UCA1 regulated cell cycle distribution via CREB through PI3-K dependent pathway in bladder carcinoma cells. *Gene,* 496, 8-16.

Yang, L. Parkin, D. Li, D. Chen, Y. & Bray, F. (2004). Estimation and projection of the national profile of cancer mortality in China: 1991–2005. *British Journal of Cancer,* 90, 2157–2166.

Ying, L. Chen, Q. Wang, Y. Zhou, Z. Huang, Y. & Qiu, F. (2012). Upregulated MALAT-1 contributes to bladder cancer cell migration by inducing epithelial-to-mesenchymal transition. *Mol Biosyst,* 9, 2289-2294.

Yutkin, V. Nisman, B. & Pode, D. (2010). Can urinary biomarkers replace cystoscopic examination in bladder cancer surveillance? *Expert Rev Anticancer Ther,* 10, 787–790.

Zhang, X. Rice, K. Wang, Y. Chen, W. Zhong, Y. Nakayama, Y. Zhou, Y. & Klibanski, A. (2010). Maternally expressed gene 3 (MEG3) noncoding ribonucleic acid: isoform structure, expression, and functions. *Endocrinology,* 151, 939-947.

Zhou, Y. Zhang, X. & Klibanski, A. (2012). MEG3 noncoding RNA: a tumor suppressor. *J Mol Endocrinol,* 48, R45-53.

In: Bladder Cancer
Editor: Samantha Haggerty
ISBN: 978-1-63321-666-2

Chapter 6

HISTOLOGICAL VARIANTS OF UROTHELIAL CARCINOMA: DIAGNOSTIC, PROGNOSTIC AND THERAPEUTIC IMPLICATIONS

Hyung Suk Kim and Ja Hyeon Ku*
Department of Urology, Seoul National University College of Medicine, Korea

ABSTRACT

The majority (more than 90%) of malignant neoplasms arising in the bladder are pure urothelial (transitional cell) carcinomas, and the rest (less than 10%) consist of histological variants of bladder cancer, including urothelial carcinoma admixed with other histologic patterns (squamous/glandular differentiation, nested, microcystic, clear cell, plasmacytoid, lymphoepithelioma-like, micropapillary, sarcomatoid variants, etc.) and pure forms of non-urothelial carcinoma (squamous cell carcinoma, adenocarcinoma, small cell carcinoma, etc.). These histological variants of bladder cancer have been described in a number of case series for several years and have been recognized in the 2004 World Health Organization Classification of urothelial cancers. These histological variants of bladder cancer have clinical significance at various levels, including diagnostic, that is, recognition of the morphological variant is necessary in order to avoid diagnostic misinterpretations; prognostic for patient risk stratification; and

* Corresponding author: Ja Hyeon Ku, M.D. PhD., Department of Urology, Seoul National University Hospital, 101 Daehak-ro, Jongno-gu, Seoul 110-744, Korea, Tel: 82-2-2072-0361, Fax: 82-2-742-4665, E-mail: kuuro70@snu.ac.kr.

therapeutic, where a diagnosis of a particular variant may be associated with the administration of a therapy distinctive from that used in conventional urothelial carcinoma. In this article, we will chiefly review the literature on the histological variants of urothelial carcinoma with a focus on the prognostic and therapeutic implications of histological variants for the management of patients with bladder cancer.

INTRODUCTION

Bladder cancer is the most common urinary tract malignant neoplasm worldwide. In the United States, the majority of bladder cancers are pure urothelial carcinomas (UC), which account for more than 90% of all bladder cancers. The remaining less than 10% of bladder cancers include UC admixed with other histological variants and non-UC. According to‘ Pathology and genetics of tumours of the urinary system and male genital organs’ in the 2004 World Health Organization (WHO) classification of tumours, these histological variants of UC consist of squamous/glandular differentiation, nested, microcystic, clear cell, plasmacytoid, lymphoepithelioma-like, micropapillary, and sarcomatoid variants (Montironi and Lopez-Beltran 2005). This classification of histological variants is based primarily on the morphologic features, but each histological variant is characterized by its distinct biological behavior. The recognition of these histological variants of urothelial neoplasia is critical because (1) some subtypes may be associated with a different clinical outcome and prognosis owing to a different propensity for stage and grade at the time of presentation, metastasis and local recurrence after treatment, (2) each subtype may respond differently to different therapeutic approaches such as transurethral resection, intravesical therapy, systemic chemotherapy, and radical cystectomy, and (3) awareness of the unusual pattern may be critical in avoiding diagnostic misinterpretations (Young and Eble 1991, Tavora and Epstein 2008, Amin 2009). In this article, we review the literature on the histological variants of UC with a focus on their prognostic and therapeutic implications.

UC WITH SQUAMOUS DIFFERENTIATION

Squamous differentiation is the most common histological variant of UC, and it is observed in 8-15% of UC invading the lamina propria and in 20-60%

of muscle invasive UC (Lopez-Beltran et al. 2007, Scosyrev et al. 2009, Shanks and Iczkowski 2009). Keratinization and/or intercellular bridges are classical morphological features characteristic of squamous differentiation (Shokeir 2004). This variant has been known to have an unfavorable prognosis in association with high grade and advanced pathologic stage disease (greater than T2, lymph node metastasis) at the time of presentation (Logothetis et al. 1988, Martin et al. 1989, Billis et al. 2001, Lopez-Beltran et al. 2007, Black et al. 2007, Erdemir et al. 2007, Antunes et al. 2007, Wasco et al. 2007, Kim et al. 2012, Mitra et al. 2014). Some case series on radical cystectomy for UC have suggested that squamous differentiation in UC was associated with higher recurrence and progression (Erdemir et al. 2007, Antunes et al. 2007), and it was an independent predictor of local recurrence and cancer specific survival on multivariate analysis (Honma et al. 2004, Antunes et al. 2007). Whereas, other studies have demonstrated that the presence of squamous differentiation did not have an effect on the disease specific survival rate (Wasco et al. 2007, Lopez-Beltran et al. 2007). Particularly, it has been reported in recent studies that after adjusting for the pathologic stage, there were no differences in survival outcomes between UC with squamous differentiation and pure UC (Kim et al. 2012, Mitra et al. 2014). Thus, the prognostic significance of squamous differentiation in UC is unclear so far. Some studies have demonstrated that patients having UC with squamous differentiation show a poor response to chemotherapy or radiation therapy, but it is unclear whether the poor response is a reflection of histology or the advanced stage of the disease (Black et al. 2009). A recent retrospective review of the Southwest Oncology Group (SWOG) database has demonstrated that the presence of squamous or glandular differentiation in locally advanced UC of the bladder does not seem to confer resistance to M-VAC (methotrexate/vinblastine/doxorubicin/cisplatin) chemotherapy, and in fact may be an indication for the use of neoadjuvant chemotherapy prior to radical cystectomy (Scosyrev et al. 2011). Pure form of squamous cell carcinoma is not more radiosensitive than UC, and it is less chemosensitive (Shokeir 2004, Lagwinski et al. 2007). Therefore, there is no good alternative for adjuvant or neoadjuvant therapy. Because of this feature, in combination with the fact that most of the patients die due to local progression, some centers recommend neoadjuvant or adjuvant radiotherapy for squamous cell carcinoma (Black et al. 2009, Pons et al. 2011). However, there is no indication that radiotherapy would offer any benefit to patients having UC with squamous differentiation. Currently, as for the pure form of squamous cell carcinoma of the bladder and conventional invasive UC, radical cystectomy is also considered as the main therapeutic approach for this histological variant (Budia Alba et al. 1999, Shokeir 2004, Lagwinski et al. 2007). In addition, there was a report demonstrating that in case of non-bulky (<4 cm), transurethrally completely resectable non-muscle invasive disease (Ta, T1), intravesical Bacillus Calmette-Guerin (BCG) therapy after transurethral resection may have an effect on the prevention of disease progression (Shapur et al. 2011). But, larger studies are required to confirm whether or not, on a stage-by-stage basis, patients with squamous differentiation have a worse prognosis than patients with pure UC. Following that, it remains to be determined whether or not these patients need different management protocols, as there have been suggestions in the literature of poor responses to chemotherapy and radiotherapy (Logothetis et al. 1988, Martin et al. 1989).

UC with Glandular Differentiation

Glandular differentiation is more infrequent than squamous differentiation, with an incidence of approximately less than 10% of UCs (Lopez-Beltran and Cheng 2006, Black et al. 2009). It is usually in the form of small tubular or gland-like spaces in UC or as a histology similar to enteric adenocarcinoma and rarely, a coexistent signet ring cell or a mucinous component may be present (Lopez-Beltran et al. 1988, Amin 2009). Patients with only glandular differentiation should be labeled as adenocarcinoma, rather than UC with glandular differentiation (Chalasani et al. 2009). Most published reports have not looked at glandular differentiation separately, but rather have combined it with squamous differentiation (Lopez-Beltran et al. 1988, Billis et al. 2001, Black et al. 2007, Erdemir et al. 2007, Wasco et al. 2007). Similar to squamous differentiation in UC, it is thought that glandular differentiation may also indicate an unfavorable prognosis, possibly due to its association with high grade and high stage UC, but this point has not been sufficiently investigated due to its rarity, and hence any definite conclusions cannot be made. The most recent studies demonstrated that although this variant was associated with a higher pathologic stage than pure UC, there were no differences in survival outcomes between UC with glandular differentiation and pure UC after adjusting for the pathologic stage (Kim et al. 2012, Mitra et al. 2014). Glandular differentiation in unresectable UC is reported to predict increased chemotherapy resistance, compared to pure UC or UC with squamous differentiation (Shanks and Iczkowski 2009). With respect to the pure form of adenocarcinoma, there was one report suggesting that adjuvant radiotherapy has been recommended, but there is no evidence that it is beneficial in UC with glandular differentiation. For transurethrally resectable non-muscle invasive tumors, intravesical BCG therapy may be effective (Shapur et al. 2011). However, to date, no consensus on the therapeutic recommendations has been made in the clinical context.

NESTED VARIANT OF UC

The nested variant of UC should be recognized as a malignant process. Approximately 60-70 cases have been reported, most as case reports (Drew et al. 1996a, Murphy and Deana 1992, Holmäng and Johansson 2001, Lin et al. 2003, Dhall et al. 2007, Neşe et al. 2007). This rare subtype of UC may sometimes be confused with von Brunn's nests, and hence, differentiation from von Brunn's nests is essential (Drew et al. 1996a, Volmar et al. 2003). Occasionally, reactive von Brunn's nests show florid proliferation, but there is absence of cytological atypia and extension of von Brunn's nests to a uniform level within the lamina propria, creating a sharp, linear border at the base (Talbert and Young 1989a, Volmar et al. 2003). On the contrary, nested variant of UC is composed of closely packed nests of small, irregularly sized and contoured cells, with unevenly distributed infiltrative patterns (detrusor muscle invasion) in spite of the bland nuclear features and subtle cytological atypia (Dhall et al. 2007). Several other tumors primarily or secondarily involving the bladder may exhibit a nested pattern, including paraganglioma, melanoma, carcinoid tumor, and prostate adenocarcinoma (Amin 2009). The diagnostic method using immunohistochemistry may be helpful in the differential diagnosis of this variant (Lin et al. 2003, Volmar et al. 2003, McKenney and Amin 2005, Zhai et al. 2007, Dhall et al. 2007). In the nested variant of UC, urothelial surface changes such as carcinoma *in situ* (CIS) are frequently absent, but lymphovascular invasion is frequent (Amin 2009). This variant is often in the advanced stage at the time of presentation despite the relatively bland cytology (Drew et al. 1996a, Holmäng and Johansson 2001, Wasco et al. 2010, Linder et al. 2013). However, it is uncertain whether the aggressive clinical behavior is independent of the stage. Data on the outcome and prognosis of nested variant of UC are limited due to the very small number of reported cases, the diverse follow-up period, different treatment strategies, and absence of prospective comparative analysis within large series of usual and unusual UC. Information from a few larger case studies on nested variant suggests that many of these patients have an aggressive clinical course characterized by progressive disease, metastasis and death underscoring the importance of recognizing this variant in limited or superficial biopsies and distinguishing it from its many benign mimics (Drew et al. 1996a, Murphy and Deana 1992, Holmäng and Johansson 2001, Lin et al. 2003, Dhall et al. 2007, Neşe et al. 2007, Nigwekar and Amin 2008). In contrast, a recent matched analysis has reported that although the nested variant was associated with a higher pathologic stage (more than T3, nodal invasion) than pure UC, there was no differences in recurrence free and cancer specific survival rates between the nested variant and pure UC after adjusting for the pathologic stage (Linder et al. 2013). There are few evidences regarding the treatment recommendations for the nested variant thus far. Analysis of a small case series demonstrated that intravesical BCG therapy after complete transurethral resection of the non-muscle invasive tumors may be effectual in preventing tumor progression (Shapur et al. 2011). However, considering the aggressive nature of this variant, the therapeutic approaches should include aggressive multimodality approaches with radical cystectomy as the mainstay of treatment (Neşe et al. 2007, Dhall et al. 2007).

Microcystic Variant of UC

UC with an inverted growth pattern may rarely have microcystic architecture, either focally or more extensively, which may lead to the diagnosis of cystitis cystica (Talbert and Young 1989b, Young and Oliva 1996). Only a small number of cases (less than 20 cases) have been described by several authors (Young and Zukerberg 1991, Leroy et al. 2002, Sari et al. 2007). The pattern is characterized by a prominent widespread numerous cystic changes within nests of UC or UC with glandular differentiation. The cysts are round to oval or slit-like, sometimes measuring 1-2 mm (Young and Zukerberg 1991). This histological variant has been mostly described in the bladder (Talbert and Young 1989b, Young and Zukerberg 1991, Young and Eble 1991, Young and Oliva 1996, Radopoulos et al. 2005) and occasionally in the upper urinary tract (Leroy et al. 2002). One study has reported a case of UC with a mainly inverted and focally microcystic growth pattern at the bladder neck/prostatic urethra involving the prostatic urethra (Shanks and Iczkowski 2009). Another study has described an extremely rare case of metastatic spread of microcystic UC to the penis (Sari et al. 2007). On the basis of the findings of several case series, although this variant is suggested to have an unfavorable prognosis in association with invasive UC (Radopoulos et al. 2005, Sari et al. 2007), there is no evident or noticeable biological significance associated with this histological variant of UC. The main differential diagnosis includes benign lesions such as cystitis cystica, cystitis glandularis, and nephrogenic adenoma, which generally have a very organized appearance and lack the overt variation in size that is typical of microcystic carcinoma (Amin 2009). Thus, the clinical importance of the microcystic variant of UC may lie in its potential to be mistaken for benign lesions (Talbert and Young 1989b, Young and Eble 1991,Young and Oliva 1996).

UC WITH CLEAR CELL FEATURES

Several reports have described UC with glycogen-rich, clear cytoplasm (Kotliar et al. 1995, Oliva et al. 2002). These carcinomas are typically high grade, and therefore the differential diagnosis is critical and includes clear cell adenocarcinoma, metastatic renal cell carcinoma, and prostate carcinoma (Amin 2009). Clear cell adenocarcinoma of the bladder is more common in females and typically shows a combination of morphological patterns within the same tumor including a solid, papillary, or tubulo-cystic architectural arrangement (Sung et al. 2008, Drew et al. 1996b). The cytoplasm may be eosinophilic or clear and the cells may have a hobnail appearance (Drew et al. 1996b, Gilcrease et al. 1998,Sung et al. 2008).Whereas, poorly differentiated UC with clear cell features have a more sheet-like growth pattern and often have more characteristic appearing areas, at least focally, of UC with conventional morphology (Kotliar et al. 1995, Oliva et al. 2002). Besides, clear cell carcinoma may be positive for cytokeratin 7 and CA 125, and sometimes for cytokeratin 20 (Oliva et al. 2002). Metastatic renal cell carcinoma to the bladder can usually be excluded on the basis of the presence of renal mass. Also, immunochemistry results such as co-expression of cytokeratin and vimentin, positivity for renal cell carcinoma antigen and PAX-2, and negative reaction for cytokeratin 7 and 20 may be helpful for making the diagnosis of metastatic renal cell carcinoma to the bladder (Sim et al. 1999, Gupta et al. 2009). Prostate carcinoma typically involves the muscularis propria and may spare the lamina propria and lining mucosa, because it directly invades the bladder wall from the prostate. Strong and diffuse immunoreactivity for prostate-specific antigen (PSA) would support the diagnosis of prostate carcinoma. The markers such as cytokeratin 7 and 20, p63, thrombomodulin, and high-molecular-weight cytokeratin, which are positive in UC, are usually negative in prostate carcinomas (Di Como et al.

2002, Parker et al. 2003, McKenney and Amin 2005). Owing to the scarcity of reported articles relevant to clear cell UC, there is no well-defined evidence with regard to its prognosis and effective therapeutic approaches. But, some data from several case series indicate that the prognosis can be determined by the stage of concomitant UC (Kotliar et al. 1995, Oliva et al. 2002).

PLASMACYTOID UC

In the recent years, UC has been reported to have a marked similarity to plasma cells (Zhang et al. 2002, Soylu et al. 2005, Coyne and Sim 2006, Kohno et al. 2006, Mai et al. 2006, Fritsche et al. 2008, Gaafar et al. 2008, Ro et al. 2008, Lopez-Beltran et al. 2009, Sato et al. 2009, Nigwekar et al. 2009, Zhang et al. 2013, Keck et al. 2013). The plasmacytoid variant is characterized by eccentrically located nuclei and discohesive cells with moderate to abundant eosinophilic cytoplasm, whose morphology closely resembles that of plasma cells (Kohno et al. 2006, Fritsche et al. 2008, Ro et al. 2008, Lopez-Beltran et al. 2009). The neoplastic cells are poorly differentiated or undifferentiated, and usually show a coexisting typical high grade UC or occasionally other histological variants such as glandular, sarcomatoid, nested, micropapillary, and sarcomatoid patterns (Gaafar et al. 2008, Lopez-Beltran et al. 2009, Nigwekar et al. 2009). A plasmacytoid histology may also be observed in a variety of bladder neoplasms, including hematopoietic tumors (malignant lymphoma, plasmacytoma) and non-hematopoietic tumors (malignant melanoma, metastatic lobular and gastric adenocarcinoma, paraganglioma, and rhabdomyosarcoma) (Kohno et al. 2006). In this setting, immunohistochemical study may be helpful in the differential diagnosis. Plasmacytoid UC shows a strong reactivity for epithelial membrane antigen such as cytokeratins 7, 20, and AE1/AE3, whereas it may be negative for vimentin, LCA, lymphoid marker (kappa/lambda light chains), E-cadherin, S-100 protein, HMB 45, Melan A, smooth muscle actin, and desmin (Lopez-Beltran et al. 2009, Nigwekar et al. 2009, Sato et al. 2009, Zhang et al. 2013). It may be also positive for CD138 (Lopez-Beltran et al. 2009). The prognosis of this histological variant, which is commonly demonstrated in the relevant case series, is uniformly poor, with most of the patients showing advanced stage with high propensity for invasion (more than invasion of lamina propria and muscularis propria), metastatic disease progression (lymph node metastasis, intraperitoneal metastasis), and high recurrence rate (Sahin et al. 1991, Kohno et al. 2006, Mai et al. 2006, Fritsche et al. 2008, Gaafar et al.

2008, Nigwekar et al. 2009, Sato et al. 2009, Lopez-Beltran et al. 2009, Ricardo-Gonzalez et al. 2012, Zhang et al. 2013, Keck et al. 2013, Dayyani et al. 2013). On account of the limited number of reported cases, it is difficult to deduce whether this poor prognosis is due to the histological pattern or because of the frequently accompanying high grade and high stage UC. Radical cystectomy is recommended as the first-line therapeutic approach for plasmacytoid UC (Soylu et al. 2005, Kohno et al. 2006, Fritsche et al. 2008, Zhang et al. 2013, Keck et al. 2013). Some literatures suggest that neoadjuvant or adjuvant chemotherapy may be effective for the management of plasmacytoid UC (Kohno et al. 2006, Fritsche et al. 2008, Keck et al. 2013). However, it has been reported that although pathological down- staging was observed in about 80% of the patients treated with neoadjuvant chemotherapy, recurrences are common and the most common site of recurrence was in the peritoneum (Dayyani et al. 2013). Thus, there is no appreciable consensus on the optimal treatment approaches for this histological variant thus far.

Lymphoepithelioma-Like Carcinoma of the Urinary Bladder

Lymphoepithelioma-like carcinoma is composed of diffuse sheets of tumor cells with a typical syncytial growth pattern (Amin et al. 1994b, Lopez-Beltrán et al. 2001). The ill-defined cell boundaries and heavy lymphoid infiltrate (mixture of B and T cells) or admixture of other inflammatory cells (plasma cells, histiocytes, and granulocytes) can cause confusion with either lymphoma or an inflammatory process such as chronic cystitis (Zukerberg et al. 1991, Amin et al. 1994b, Holmang et al. 1998). Tumors with these histological features are so named due to their remarkable similarity to the lymphoepithelioma of the nasopharynx (Amin et al. 1994b, Gulley et al. 1995, Holmang et al. 1998, Lopez-Beltrán et al. 2001, Tamas et al. 2007).They have also been reported at other sites, including the prostate, breast, cervix, skin, lung, thymus, stomach, and salivary glands (Amin et al. 1994b). The incidence of this histologic variant is 0.4%–1.3% of all bladder carcinomas, the mean age at diagnosis is 60 years, and there is male predominance (in approximately 70% of cases reported in literature) (Holmang et al. 1998, Lopez-Beltrán et al. 2001, Porcaro et al. 2003). Unlike lymphoepithelioma-like carcinoma at other sites (esp. nasopharynx), relationship with Epstein-Barr virus (by immunohistochemistry and in situ hybridization) has not been identified

(Gulley et al. 1995, Izquierdo-García et al. 2004, Lopez-Beltrán et al. 2001, Tamas et al. 2007). Histologically, the syncytial arrangement and typical cytology are essential for the diagnosis of lymphoepithelioma-like carcinoma (Amin et al. 1994b, Gulley et al. 1995, Fadare et al. 2009). Immunohistochemical study shows a reactivity against epithelial membrane antigen (CKs; AE1/AE3, AE1, AE3, CK7, and CK8) and several cytokeratins (CK20, CD44v6) (Lopez-Beltrán et al. 2001). Besides, the frequent presence of UroVysion FISH abnormalities, urothelial CIS, and p53 positivity by immunohistochemistry suggest a similar pathogenesis to high-grade invasive UC (Williamson et al. 2011). According to the proportion of lymphoepithelioma component, this subtype of UC is classified into focal (<50%), predominant (>50%), and pure (100%) (Zukerberg et al. 1991, Amin et al. 1994b). One study demonstrated that approximately 57% of cases were pure, and the rest (43%) were mixed form with urothelial or non-urothelial element (adenocarcinoma, squamous carcinoma) (Tamas et al. 2007). Although the majority of reported tumors are in the advanced stage (greater than the T2 stage) at presentation (Holmang et al. 1998, Lopez-Beltrán et al. 2001, Tamas et al. 2007) and reported rates of metastasis range from 12% to 15% (Tamas et al. 2007), this histological variant may be associated with a favorable prognosis, if these tumors are of the pure or predominant type rather than the focal type (Holmang et al. 1998, Lopez-Beltrán et al. 2001, Porcaro et al. 2003, Williamson et al. 2011). Similar to the other variants of UC, there are no obvious guidelines for the treatment of lymphoepithelioma-like carcinoma. However, several case series demonstrate that the pure or predominant type of tumors respond better to chemotherapy as the primary treatment modality than conventional UC, providing a better potential to salvage bladder function (Amin et al. 1994b, Holmang et al. 1998, Porcaro et al. 2003, Williamson et al. 2011); and this advantage may be lost when the urothelial elements predominate (Lopez-Beltrán et al. 2001). In one large case series, cases treated with cystectomy showed a 5-year actuarial recurrence-free risk of 59% (62 and 57%, for pure and mixed cases, respectively), which was similar to the 5-year recurrence free rate of 65-68% in cases of muscle-invasive bladder cancer treated by cystectomy. Lymphoepithelioma-like carcinoma, whether in pure or mixed form, has a similar prognosis to conventional UC when treated by cystectomy (Tamas et al. 2007).

MICROPAPILLARY UC

Micropapillary variant of UC is another highly malignant histologic subtype displaying the micropapillary architecture, which is similar to that of serous ovarian carcinoma (Amin et al. 1994a, Johansson et al. 1999, Samaratunga and Khoo 2004, Alvarado-Cabrero et al. 2005). Relevant case series have consistently reported this variant, and have presented an incidence of 0.6-1% of UCs, definite male predominance, and a mean age of between 65 and 70 years (Amin et al. 1994a, Johansson et al. 1999, Samaratunga and Khoo 2004, Alvarado-Cabrero et al. 2005, Kamat et al. 2006, Kamat et al. 2007, Wang et al. 2012). In the majority of the reported cases, micropapillary UC originates from the urinary bladder, but it can also occur in the upper urinary tract (Vang and Abrams 2000, Holmang et al. 2006, Perez-Montiel et al. 2006, Munakata et al. 2007, Guo et al. 2009). The micropapillary component may be discovered in the non-invasive component, invasive component, and in metastatic sites. Histologically, in the non-invasive component, it forms slender, delicate filiform processes or small papillary clusters of tumor cells, whereas in the invasive component or in metastatic sites, it is composed of infiltrating tight clusters of micropapillary aggregates that are often present within the lacunae (Amin et al. 1994a). Unlike in an ovarian papillary serous carcinoma, Psammoma bodies are very rarely observed (Amin et al. 1994a). According to the proportion of the micropapillary component within the tumors, it can be classified as focal (<10%), moderate (10-49%), and extensive (50-100%). It has been generally demonstrated that the more is the percentage of the micropapillary component in the tumors, the worse are its clinical outcome and prognosis (Amin et al. 1994a, Samaratunga and Khoo 2004, Alvarado-Cabrero et al. 2005, Compérat et al. 2010), and even the focal component has been associated with an adverse prognosis (Samaratunga and Khoo 2004, Compérat et al. 2010). This variant mainly occurs in association with conventional UC, and in extremely rare cases, other histologic patterns such as adenocarcinoma, UC admixed with squamous, or glandular differentiation are observed (Johansson et al. 1999, Samaratunga and Khoo 2004, Lopez-Beltran et al. 2010). The neoplasm showing micropapillary features may also be observed in other primary sites such as lung, breast, pancreas, kidney, and salivary glands (Amin 2009, Shanks and Iczkowski 2009). In this instance, the bladder may be considered as the primary origin site of micropapillary carcinoma if there is no obvious primary tumor at another site on clinical and radiographic evaluation. Because distant metastasis usually shows the same micropapillary morphology, the likelihood of UC as the site of primary origin should be considered if the micropapillary component is seen in the peritoneum, abdominal lymph nodes or mesentery of a male patient with unknown primary site or in a female with normal appearing ovaries (Amin 2009, Shanks and Iczkowski 2009, Pons et al. 2011). Identification of an admixed UC with a more typical morphology or immunohistochemical results (CK20, CK7 and uroplakin III positivity) may be helpful (Maranchie et al. 2000, Samaratunga and Khoo 2004, Munakata et al. 2007). The micropapillary UC is usually high grade, in the advanced stage (more than T2 stage), and has a high DNA index at the time of presentation (Amin et al. 1994a, Johansson et al. 1999, Samaratunga and Khoo 2004, Alvarado-Cabrero et al. 2005, Kamat et al. 2006, Kamat et al. 2007, Compérat et al. 2010, Lopez-Beltran et al. 2010, Wang et al. 2012, Wang and Wang 2013). Also, urothelial CIS is present in more than 50% of cases, and the same micropapillary pattern and lymphovascular invasion is observed in more than 50% of cases (Amin et al. 1994a, Samaratunga and Khoo 2004, Alvarado-Cabrero et al. 2005, Holmang et al. 2006, Kamat et al. 2007, Compérat et al. 2010). Lymph node involvement and distant metastasis are commonly observed at presentation, and they are detected in approximately 47% and 35% of cases, respectively (Compérat et al. 2010). Thus, micropapillary UC has a highly aggressive behavior and shows a poorer prognosis than conventional UC (Alvarado-Cabrero et al. 2005, Lopez-Beltran et al. 2010, Wang et al. 2012,Wang and Wang 2013). It has been reported that the 5-year and 10-year overall survival rates of the patients with micropapillary UC were 51 and 24%, respectively (Kamat et al. 2007) and the 3-year disease-specific survival rate for patients with MPUC was 39.5%, whereas that for the patients with pure UC was 55.3% (Alvarado-Cabrero et al. 2005). However, other recent studies demonstrated that there were no differences in survival outcomes between micropapillary variant and pure UC after controlling for the pathologic stage (Wang et al. 2012, Fairey et al. 2014). Owing to high correlation of micropapillary UC with muscle-invasive disease (greater than the T2 stage), it has been suggested that if there is no muscle layer in the initial biopsy, re-biopsy including the detrusor muscle should be performed for the accurate evaluation of staging (Amin et al. 1994a, Alvarado-Cabrero et al. 2005). Adjuvant chemotherapy with the M-VAC regimen seems to be ineffective for this variant (Heudel et al. 2009). Several reports have demonstrated that although non-muscle invasive micropapillary UC was identified in a transurethral resection specimen, disease progression (T2 or greater) in about 67% of patients after intravesical therapy with BCG (Kamat et al. 2006, Kamat et al. 2007), upstaging of the micropapillary component (79% of cases) and primary tumor stage in the final cystectomy specimen were observed (Compérat et al. 2010). Besides, patients treated with preoperative chemotherapy followed by cystectomy showed an equivalent overall survival rate compared to those treated with cystectomy only (Kamat et al. 2007). Therefore, it is suggested that intravesical BCG therapy appears to be ineffective against micropapillary UC and immediate cystectomy should be considered for the management of micropapillary UC, regardless of the proportion of the micropapillary component within the tumor and primary tumor stage at initial diagnosis (Kamat et al. 2006, Kamat et al. 2007, Perepletchikov and Parwani 2009).On the other hand, due to the high risk of relapse of this variant, neoadjuvant chemotherapy is recommended (Black et al. 2009).

SARCOMATOID VARIANT OF UC

Sarcomatoid variant of UC is an uncommon malignant neoplasm with biphasic morphology exhibiting both epithelial and mesenchymal elements, and it includes carcinosarcoma (carcinoma with true sarcomatous components) and sarcomatoid carcinoma (carcinoma with mesenchymal-appearing spindle cell component) (Lopez-Beltran et al. 1998, Jones and Young 1997, Omeroglu et al. 2002, Ogishima et al. 2002, Sung et al. 2007, Wright et al. 2007, Wang et al. 2010). The reported incidence ranges from 0.2% to 4.3% (Torenbeek et al. 1994, Wright et al. 2007, Chalasani et al. 2009, Wang et al. 2010,Pons et al. 2011). The clinical usefulness of this distinction between the 2 tumor types is controversial (Wick and Swanson 1993, Reuter 1993, Eble et al. 2004). Recently, there is an emerging consensus that sarcomatoid carcinoma is the most appropriate term for these neoplasms. The latest WHO classification has applied this term to all tumors showing morphologic and/or immunologic evidence of both malignant epithelial and mesenchymal differentiation (Wick and Swanson 1993, Reuter 1993, Eble et al. 2004, Montironi and Lopez-Beltran 2005). Several molecular genetic studies have suggested a common clonal origin for the carcinomatous and sarcomatous components, and hence, the outcome of tumors with and without heterogeneous elements may be usually similar (Sung et al. 2007, Armstrong et al. 2009, Cheng et al. 2011). However, a recent study conducted using the Surveillance, Epidemiology, and End Results (SEER) database (Wright et al. 2007) demonstrated that sarcomatoid carcinoma and carcinosarcoma presented at a higher T stage and more frequently with locally advanced and distant metastases compared to

UC; but when separated, the overall mortality was worse in patients with carcinosarcoma than in those with sarcomatoid carcinoma, which indicates that there is some value to the clinical distinction between the two types. The sarcomatoid areas may merge with foci of UC, squamous cell carcinoma, adenocarcinoma or small cell carcinoma (Ishida et al. 2013). Also, in a decreasing order of frequency, areas of osteosarcoma, chondrosarcoma, rhabdomyosarcoma, liposarcoma, angiosarcoma, or a mixture of sarcoma histologies may be seen (Reuter 1993). The differential diagnosis includes benign conditions such as pseudosarcomatous myofibroblastic proliferation (PMP) of the bladder and malignancies such as UC with chondroid or osseous metaplasia, primary sarcomas, chiefly leiomyosarcoma (Harik et al. 2006, Westfall et al. 2009). Morphologically, more myxoid and hypocellular regions toward the surface, greater cellularity with a fibrous background toward the base, 'nodular fascitis' type appearance of the lesion, the absence of epithelial component and nuclear atypia, which are the features observed in PMP, are important for making a distinction from a malignant process (Harik et al. 2006). Immunohistochemical study may also be helpful in the differential diagnosis of the sarcomatoid lesion of the bladder. Sarcomatoid carcinomas may be distinguished from PMP and leiomyosarcoma by their positive reactivity for p63, CK5/6, and high-molecular-weight cytokeratin, since PMP and leiomyosarcoma show negativity for p63, CK5/6, and high-molecular-weight cytokeratin (Westfall et al. 2009, McKenney and Amin 2005). Compared to conventional UC, nearly all sarcomatoid carcinomas present at a higher stage and grade, frequently with lymph node and distant metastases, and have an extremely aggressive clinical course resulting in a very poor prognosis, even after adjusting for the stage (Torenbeek et al. 1994, Lopez-Beltran et al. 1998, Ikegami et al. 2000, Ogishima et al. 2002, Wright et al. 2007, Wang et al. 2010). An estimated 70% of patients die within 2 years from the initial diagnosis (Reuter 1993, Torenbeek et al. 1994, Jones and Young 1997, Lopez-Beltran et al. 1998, Ikegami et al. 2000, Sung et al. 2007, Wright et al. 2007). There is no standardized clinical management protocol for this variant. It has been described that in case of non-muscle invasive sarcomatoid UC, intravesical BCG therapy following complete transurethral resection may be ineffective for the prevention of disease progression (Shapur et al. 2011). Likewise, one group has suggested radical cystectomy as the preferred option for patients with T1 disease, rather than intravesical therapy (Black et al. 2007, Black et al. 2009). Even though it was a small case series, it has been reported that almost half (45%) of 11 patients who received neoadjuvant chemotherapy for clinical T2 and T3 tumors were down-staged to T0 on the cystectomy specimen (Black et al. 2009). Given that this variant has an aggressive clinical course, aggressive multimodality treatment approaches including neoadjuvant or adjuvant chemotherapy, radiotherapy, and radical cystectomy with pelvic lymph node dissection would be probably required for the management of this disease, which are applied equally to high grade conventional UC with similar degrees of invasion. Some of the authors have suggested application of the treatment paradigms used for other solid tumors with similar histological features, such as uterus or lung carcinosarcoma (Wright et al. 2007).

CONCLUSION

Compared to conventional UC, the histological variants of UC usually show a high grade and a high stage at presentation, and hence, there may be an increase in the possibility of locally advanced disease and metastasis. Occasionally, each variant can occur in combination with another histological variant other than UC. It is crucial to distinguish them from the primary or secondary bladder lesions. Although these variants usually present in an advanced stage, their prognostic implications may be variable depending on their histopathological features. It seems that 1) the prognosis of plasmacytoid, micropapillary, and sarcomatoid variants is worse than that of UC, 2) lymphoepithelioma-like carcinomas may show a better prognosis due to their chemosensitivity, 3) squamous/glandular differentiation, nested, microcystic, and clear cell variants do not show a definite prognosis. However, it is not completely understood whether prognosis of these histological variants is independent of the pathologic stage. A consensus on the definite treatment guidelines for each histologic variant has not been reached as yet owing to their infrequent incidence and application of different treatment strategies from institution to institution. Therefore, further, multicentric, prospective researches would be required to clarify the prognosis and establish a tailored treatment protocol for each histological variant of UC.

REFERENCES

Alvarado-Cabrero, I., Sierra-Santiesteban, F. I., Mantilla-Morales, A. & Hernandez-Hernandez, D. M. (2005). Micropapillary carcinoma of the urothelial tract. A clinicopathologic study of 38 cases. *Ann Diagn Pathol*, Feb. *9*, 1-5.

Amin, M. B. (2009). Histological variants of urothelial carcinoma: diagnostic, therapeutic and prognostic implications. *Modern Pathology*, *22*, S96-S118.

Amin, M. B., Ro, J. Y., El-Sharkawy, T., Lee, K. M., Troncoso, P., Silva, E. G., Ord Ez, N. G. & Ayala, A. G. (1994a). Micropapillary Variant of Transitional Cell Carcinoma of the Urinary Bladder Histologic Pattern Resembling Ovarian Papillary Serous Carcinoma. *The American journal of surgical pathology*, *18*, 1224-1232.

Amin, M. B., Ro, J. Y., Lee, K. M., Ord Ez, N. G., Dinney, C. P., Gulley, M. L. & Ayala, A. G. (1994b). Lymphoepithelioma-like carcinoma of the urinary bladder. *The American journal of surgical pathology*, *18*, 466-473.

Antunes, A. A., Nesrallah, L. J., Dall'oglio, M. F., Maluf, C. E., Camara, C., Leite, K. R. & Srougi, M. (2007). The role of squamous differentiation in patients with transitional cell carcinoma of the bladder treated with radical cystectomy. *International braz j urol*, 33, 339-346.

Armstrong, A. B., Wang, M., Eble, J. N., Maclennan, G. T., Montironi, R., Tan, P. -H., Lopez-Beltran, A., Zhang, S., Baldridge, L. A. & Spartz, H. (2009). TP53 mutational analysis supports monoclonal origin of biphasic sarcomatoid urothelial carcinoma (carcinosarcoma) of the urinary bladder. *Modern Pathology*, *22*, 113-118.

Billis, A., Schenka, A. A., Ramos, C. C., Carneiro, L. T. & Ara Jo, V. (2001). Squamous and/or glandular differentiation in urothelial carcinoma, prevalence and significance in transurethral resections of the bladder. *International urology and nephrology*, *33*, 631-633.

Black, P. C., Brown, G. A. & Dinney, C. P. (2007). *Clinical and therapeutic significance of aberrant differentiation patterns in bladder cancer.*

Black, P. C., Brown, G. A. & Dinney, C. P. (2009). The impact of variant histology on the outcome of bladder cancer treated with curative intent. *Urologic Oncology: Seminars and Original Investigations*, 3-7. Elsevier.

Budia Alba, A., Queipo Zaragoza, J. A., Perez Ebri, M. L., Fuster Escriva, A., Vera Donoso, D. C., Vera Sempere, F. J. & Jimenez Cruz, J. F. (1999). [Comparative study of pure epidermoid carcinoma of the bladder and transitional cell carcinoma with squamous or mixed differentiated foci]. *Actas urologicas espanolas*, Feb. 23, 111-118.

Chalasani, V., Chin, J. L. & Izawa, J. I. (2009). Histologic variants of urothelial bladder cancer and nonurothelial histology in bladder cancer. *Canadian Urological Association Journal*, *3*, S193.

Cheng, L., Zhang, S., Alexander, R., Maclennan, G. T., Hodges, K. B., Harrison, B. T., Lopez-Beltran, A. & Montironi, R. (2011). Sarcomatoid carcinoma of the urinary bladder: the final common pathway of urothelial carcinoma dedifferentiation. *The American journal of surgical pathology*, *35*, e34-e46.

Comp Rat, E., Roupret, M., Yaxley, J., Reynolds, J., Varinot, J., Ouza D, I., Cussenot, O. & Samaratunga, H. (2010). Micropapillary urothelial carcinoma of the urinary bladder: a clinicopathological analysis of 72 cases. *Pathology*, *42*, 650-654.

Coyne, J. D. & Sim, E. (2006). Urothelial neoplasia with plasmacytoid morphology. *Histopathology*, Jan. *48*, 200-201.

Dayyani, F., Czerniak, B. A., Sircar, K., Munsell, M. F., Millikan, R. E., Dinney, C. P. & Siefker-Radtke, A. O. (2013). Plasmacytoid urothelial carcinoma, a chemosensitive cancer with poor prognosis, and peritoneal carcinomatosis. *The Journal of urology*, *189*, 1656-1661.

Dhall, D., Al-Ahmadie, H. & Olgac, S. (2007). Nested variant of urothelial carcinoma. *Archives of pathology & laboratory medicine*, *131*, 1725-1727.

Di Como, C. J., Urist, M. J., Babayan, I., Drobnjak, M., Hedvat, C. V., Teruya-Feldstein, J., Pohar, K., Hoos, A. & Cordon-Cardo, C. (2002). p63 expression profiles in human normal and tumor tissues. *Clinical Cancer Research*, *8*, 494-501.

Drew, P. A., Furman, J., Civantos, F. & Murphy, W. M. (1996a). The nested variant of transitional cell carcinoma: an aggressive neoplasm with innocuous histology. Modern pathology: an official journal of the United States and Canadian Academy of Pathology, Inc, *9*, 989-994.

Drew, P. A., Murphy, W. M., Civantos, F. & Speights, V. (1996b). The histogenesis of clear cell adenocarcinoma of the lower urinary tract, case series and review of the literature. *Human pathology*, *27*, 248-252.

Eble, J., Sauter, G., Epstein, J. & Sesterhenn, I. (2004). Tumours of the urinary system and male genital organs: pathology and genetics. World Health Organization Classification of Tumours. Lyon.

Erdemir, F., Tunc, M., Ozcan, F., Parlaktas, B. S., Uluocak, N., Kılıcaslan, I. & Gokce, O. (2007). The effect of squamous and/or glandular differentiation on recurrence, progression and survival in urothelial carcinoma of bladder. *International urology and nephrology*, *39*, 803-807.

Fadare, O., Renshaw, I. L. & Rubin, C. (2009). Pleomorphic lymphoepithelioma-like carcinoma of the urinary bladder. *International journal of clinical and experimental pathology*, *2*, 194.

Fairey, A. S., Daneshmand, S., Wang, L., Schuckman, A., Lieskovsky, G., Djaladat, H., Cai, J., Miranda, G. & Skinner, E. C. (2014). Impact of micropapillary urothelial carcinoma variant histology on survival after radical cystectomy. *Urologic Oncology: Seminars and Original Investigations*, 110-116. Elsevier.

Fritsche, H. M., Burger, M., Denzinger, S., Legal, W., Goebell, P. J. & Hartmann, A. (2008). Plasmacytoid urothelial carcinoma of the bladder: histological and clinical features of 5 cases. *The Journal of urology*, Nov. *180*, 1923-1927.

Gaafar, A., Garmendia, M., De Miguel, E., Velasco, V., Ugalde, A., Bilbao, F. J., De Petris, G. & Lopez, J. I. (2008). [Plasmacytoid urothelial carcinoma of the urinary bladder. A study of 7 cases]. *Actas urologicas espanolas, Sep. 32*, 806-810.

Gilcrease, M. Z., Delgado, R., Vuitch, F. & Albores-Saavedra, J. (1998). Clear cell adenocarcinoma and nephrogenic adenoma of the urethra and urinary bladder: a histopathologic and immunohistochemical comparison. *Human pathology*, 29, 1451-1456.

Gulley, M. L., Amin, M. B., Nicholls, J. M., Banks, P. M., Ayala, A. G., Srigley, J. R., Eagan, P. A. & Ro, J. Y. (1995). Epstein-Barr virus is detected in undifferentiated nasopharyngeal carcinoma but not in lymphoepithelioma-like carcinoma of the urinary bladder. *Hum Pathol*, Nov. *26*, 1207-1214.

Guo, C. C., Tamboli, P. & Czerniak, B. (2009). Micropapillary variant of urothelial carcinoma in the upper urinary tract: a clinicopathologic study of 11 cases. *Archives of pathology & laboratory medicine*, *133*, 62-66.

Gupta, R., Balzer, B., Picken, M., Osunkoya, A. O., Shet, T., Alsabeh, R., Luthringer, D., Paner, G. P. & Amin, M. B. (2009). Diagnostic implications of transcription factor Pax 2 protein and transmembrane enzyme complex carbonic anhydrase IX immunoreactivity in adult renal epithelial neoplasms. *The American journal of surgical pathology*, *33*, 241-247.

Harik, L. R., Merino, C., Coindre, J. -M., Amin, M. B., Pedeutour, F. & Weiss, S. W. (2006). Pseudosarcomatous myofibroblastic proliferations of the bladder: a clinicopathologic study of 42 cases. *The American journal of surgical pathology*, *30*, 787-794.

Heudel, P., El Karak, F., Ismaili, N., Droz, J. -P. & Flechon, A. (2009). Micropapillary bladder cancer, a review of Leon Berard Cancer Center experience. *BMC urology*, *9*, 5.

Holm Ng, S. & Johansson, S. L. (2001). The nested variant of transitional cell carcinoma-a rare neoplasm with poor prognosis. *Scandinavian journal of urology and nephrology*, *35*, 102-105.

Holmang, S., Borghede, G. & Johansson, S. L. (1998). Bladder carcinoma with lymphoepithelioma-like differentiation: a report of 9 cases. *The Journal of urology*, Mar. *159*, 779-782.

Holmang, S., Thomsen, J. & Johansson, S. L. (2006). Micropapillary carcinoma of the renal pelvis and ureter. *The Journal of urology*, Feb. *175*, 463-466; discussion 466-467.

Honma, I., Masumori, N., Sato, E., Takayanagi, A., Takahashi, A., Itoh, N., Tamagawa, M., Sato, M.-A. & Tsukamoto, T. (2004). Local recurrence after radical cystectomy for invasive bladder cancer, an analysis of predictive factors. *Urology*, *64*, 744-748.

Ikegami, H., Iwasaki, H., Ohjimi, Y., Takeuchi, T., Ariyoshi, A. & Kikuchi, M. (2000). Sarcomatoid carcinoma of the urinary bladder: a clinicopathologic and immunohistochemical analysis of 14 patients. *Human pathology*, 31, 332-340.

Ishida, M., Iwai, M., Yoshida, K., Kagotani, A. & Okabe, H. (2013). Sarcomatoid carcinoma with small cell carcinoma component of the urinary bladder: A case report with review of the literature. *International journal of clinical and experimental pathology*, *6*, 1671.

Izquierdo-Garc A, F. M., Garc A-D Ez, F., Fern Ndez, I., P Rez-Rosado, A., S Ez, A., Su Rez-Vilela, D., Guerreiro-Gonz Lez, R. & Ben Itez-Alvarez, M. (2004). Lymphoepithelioma-like carcinoma of the bladder: three cases with clinicopathological and p53 protein expression study. *Virchows Archiv*, *444*, 420-425.

Johansson, S., Borghede, G. & Holmang, S. (1999). Micropapillary bladder carcinoma: a clinicopathological study of 20 cases. *The Journal of urology*, *161*, 1798-1802.

Jones, E. C. & Young, R. H. (1997). Myxoid and sclerosing sarcomatoid transitional cell carcinoma of the urinary bladder: a clinicopathologic and immunohistochemical study of 25 cases. Modern pathology: an official journal of the United States and Canadian Academy of Pathology, *Inc*, *10*, 908-916.

Kamat, A. M., Dinney, C. P., Gee, J. R., Grossman, H. B., Siefker-Radtke, A. O., Tamboli, P., Detry, M. A., Robinson, T. L. & Pisters, L. L. (2007). Micropapillary bladder cancer: a review of the University of Texas M. D. Anderson Cancer Center experience with 100 consecutive patients. *Cancer*, Jul 1. *110*, 62-67.

Kamat, A. M., Gee, J. R., Dinney, C. P., Grossman, H. B., Swanson, D. A., Millikan, R. E., Detry, M. A., Robinson, T. L. & Pisters, L. L. (2006). The case for early cystectomy in the treatment of nonmuscle invasive micropapillary bladder carcinoma. *The Journal of urology*, *175*, 881-885.

Keck, B., Wach, S., Stoehr, R., Kunath, F., Bertz, S., Lehmann, J., Stockle, M., Taubert, H., Wullich, B. & Hartmann, A. (2013). Plasmacytoid variant of bladder cancer defines patients with poor prognosis if treated with cystectomy and adjuvant cisplatin-based chemotherapy. *BMC cancer*, *13*, 71.

Kim, S. P., Frank, I., Cheville, J. C., Thompson, R. H., Weight, C. J., Thapa, P. & Boorjian, S. A. (2012). The impact of squamous and glandular differentiation on survival after radical cystectomy for urothelial carcinoma. *The Journal of urology*, *188*, 405-409.

Kohno, T., Kitamura, M., Akai, H., Takaha, M., Kawahara, K. & Oka, T. (2006). Plasmacytoid urothelial carcinoma of the bladder. *International journal of urology*, *13*, 485-486.

Kotliar, S. N., Wood, C. G., Schaeffer, A. J. & Oyasu, R. (1995). Transitional cell carcinoma exhibiting clear cell features. A differential diagnosis for clear cell adenocarcinoma of the urinary tract. *Archives of pathology & laboratory medicine*, *119*, 79-81.

Lagwinski, N., Thomas, A., Stephenson, A. J., Campbell, S., Hoschar, A. P., El-Gabry, E., Dreicer, R. & Hansel, D. E. (2007). Squamous cell carcinoma of the bladder: a clinicopathologic analysis of 45 cases. *The American journal of surgical pathology*, *31*, 1777-1787.

Leroy, X., Leteurtre, E., De La Taille, A., Augusto, D., Biserte, J. & Gosselin, B. (2002). Microcystic transitional cell carcinoma: a report of 2 cases arising in the renal pelvis. *Archives of pathology & laboratory medicine*, *126*, 859-861.

Lin, O., Cardillo, M., Dalbagni, G., Linkov, I., Hutchinson, B. & Reuter, V. E. (2003). Nested variant of urothelial carcinoma: a clinicopathologic and immunohistochemical study of 12 cases. *Modern pathology*, 16, 1289-1298.

Linder, B. J., Frank, I., Cheville, J. C., Thompson, R. H., Thapa, P., Tarrell, R. F. & Boorjian, S. A. (2013). Outcomes following radical cystectomy for nested variant of urothelial carcinoma: a matched cohort analysis. *The Journal of urology*, *189*, 1670-1675.

Logothetis, C. J., Johnson, D., Chong, C., Dexeus, F., Sella, A., Ogden, S., Smith, T., Swanson, D., Babaian, R. & Wishnow, K. (1988). Adjuvant cyclophosphamide, doxorubicin, and cisplatin chemotherapy for bladder cancer: an update. *Journal of Clinical Oncology*, *6*, 1590-1596.

Lopez-Beltr N, A., Luque, R. J., Vicioso, L., Anglada, F., Requena, M. J., Quintero, A. & Montironi, R. (2001). Lymphoepithelioma-like carcinoma of the urinary bladder: a clinicopathologic study of 13 cases. *Virchows Archiv*, *438*, 552-557.

Lopez-Beltran, A. & Cheng, L. (2006). Histologic variants of urothelial carcinoma: differential diagnosis and clinical implications. *Human pathology*, *37*, 1371-1388.

Lopez-Beltran, A., Martin, J., Garcia, J. & Toro, M. (1988). Squamous and glandular differentiation in urothelial bladder carcinomas. *Histopathology*, histochemistry and immunohistochemical expression of carcinoembryonic antigen. Histology and *histopathology*, Jan. *3*, 63-68.

Lopez-Beltran, A., Montironi, R., Blanca, A. & Cheng, L. (2010). Invasive micropapillary urothelial carcinoma of the bladder. *Human pathology*, *41*, 1159-1164.

Lopez-Beltran, A., Pacelli, A., Rothenberg, H., Wollan, P., Zincke, H., Blute, M. & Bostwick, D. (1998). Carcinosarcoma and sarcomatoid carcinoma of the bladder: clinicopathological study of 41 cases. *The Journal of urology*, *159*, 1497-1503.

Lopez-Beltran, A., Requena, M. J., Alvarez-Kindelan, J., Quintero, A., Blanca, A. & Montironi, R. (2007). Squamous differentiation in primary urothelial carcinoma of the urinary tract as seen by MAC387 immunohistochemistry. *J Clin Pathol*, Mar. *60*, 332-335.

Lopez-Beltran, A., Requena, M. J., Montironi, R., Blanca, A. & Cheng, L. (2009). Plasmacytoid urothelial carcinoma of the bladder. *Human pathology*, *40*, 1023-1028.

Mai, K. T., Park, P. C., Yazdi, H. M., Saltel, E., Erdogan, S., Stinson, W. A., Cagiannos, I. & Morash, C. (2006). Plasmacytoid urothelial carcinoma of the urinary bladder: report of seven new cases. *European urology*, *50*, 1111-1114.

Maranchie, J. K., Bouyounes, B. T., Zhang, P. L., O'donnell, M. A., Summerhayes, I. C. & De Wolf, W. C. (2000). Clinical and pathological characteristics of micropapillary transitional cell carcinoma, a highly aggressive variant. *The Journal of urology*, *163*, 748-751.

Martin, J., Jenkins, B., Zuk, R., Blandy, J. & Baithun, S. (1989). Clinical importance of squamous metaplasia in invasive transitional cell carcinoma of the bladder. *Journal of clinical pathology*, *42*, 250-253.

Mckenney, J. K. & Amin, M. B. (2005). The role of immunohistochemistry in the diagnosis of urinary bladder neoplasms. *Seminars in diagnostic pathology*, Feb. *22*, 69-87.

Mitra, A. P., Bartsch, C. C., Bartsch Jr, G., Miranda, G., Skinner, E. C. & Daneshmand, S. (2014). Does presence of squamous and glandular differentiation in urothelial carcinoma of the bladder at cystectomy portend poor prognosis? An intensive case-control analysis. *Urologic Oncology: Seminars and Original Investigations*, 117-127. Elsevier.

Montironi, R. & Lopez-Beltran, A. (2005). The 2004 WHO classification of bladder tumors: a summary and commentary. *International journal of surgical pathology*, *13*, 143-153.

Munakata, S., Tahara, H., Kojima, K. & Kishimoto, T. (2007). Micropapillary urothelial carcinoma of the renal pelvis: report of a case and review of the literature. *Medical science monitor: international medical journal of experimental and clinical research*, Apr. *13*, CS47-52.

Murphy, W. & Deana, D. (1992). The nested variant of transitional cell carcinoma: a neoplasm resembling proliferation of Brunn's nests. *Modern pathology: an official journal of the United States and Canadian Academy of Pathology, Inc*, 5, 240-243.

Neşe, N., Kandiloğlu, A. R. & Ates I, Y. Z. (2007). Nested variant of transitional cell carcinoma with osseous metaplasia of the urinary bladder: a case report and review of published reports. *International journal of urology*, *14*, 365-367.

Nigwekar, P. & Amin, M. B. (2008). The many faces of urothelial carcinoma: an update with an emphasis on recently described variants. *Advances in anatomic pathology*, Jul. *15*, 218-233.

Nigwekar, P., Tamboli, P., Amin, M. B., Osunkoya, A. O., Ben-Dor, D. & Amin, M. B. (2009). Plasmacytoid urothelial carcinoma: detailed analysis of morphology with clinicopathologic correlation in 17 cases. *The American journal of surgical pathology*, *33*, 417-424.

Ogishima, T., Kawachi, Y., Saito, A., Suzuki, F., Ishi, K. & Tanaka, T. (2002). Sarcomatoid carcinoma and carcinosarcoma of the urinary bladder. *International journal of urology*, *9*, 354-358.

Oliva, E., Amin, M. B., Jimenez, R. & Young, R. H. (2002). Clear cell carcinoma of the urinary bladder: a report and comparison of four tumors of mullerian origin and nine of probable urothelial origin with discussion of histogenesis and diagnostic problems. *The American journal of surgical pathology*, *26*, 190-197.

Omeroglu, A., Paner, G. P., Wojcik, E. M. & Siziopikou, K. (2002). A carcinosarcoma/sarcomatoid carcinoma arising in a urinary bladder diverticulum. *Archives of pathology & laboratory medicine*, *126*, 853-855.

Parker, D. C., Folpe, A. L., Bell, J., Oliva, E., Young, R. H., Cohen, C. & Amin, M. B. (2003). Potential utility of uroplakin III, thrombomodulin, high molecular weight cytokeratin, and cytokeratin 20 in noninvasive, invasive, and metastatic urothelial (transitional cell) carcinomas. *The American journal of surgical pathology*, *27*, 1-10.

Perepletchikov, A. M. & Parwani, A. V. (2009). Micropapillary urothelial carcinoma: clinico-pathologic review. *Pathology-Research and Practice*, *205*, 807-810.

Perez-Montiel, D., Hes, O., Michal, M. & Suster, S. (2006). Micropapillary Urothelial Carcinoma of the Upper Urinary Tract Clinicopathologic Study of Five Cases. *American journal of clinical pathology*, *126*, 86-92.

Pons, F., Orsola, A., Morote, J. & Bellmunt, J. (2011). Variant forms of bladder cancer: basic considerations on treatment approaches. *Current oncology reports*, *13*, 216-221.

Porcaro, A. B., Gilioli, E., Migliorini, F., Antoniolli, S. Z., Iannucci, A. & Comunale, L. (2003). Primary lymphoepithelioma-like carcinoma of the urinary bladder: report of one case with review and update of the literature after a pooled analysis of 43 patients. *International urology and nephrology*, *35*, 99-106.

Radopoulos, D., Kalyvas, K., Kotakidou, R., Panagiotopoulou, K., Katsikas, V. & Papathanasiou, M. (2005). Case report, microcystic transitional cell carcinoma of the urinary bladder. *International urology and nephrology*, *37*, 291-293.

Reuter, V. (1993). Sarcomatoid lesions of the urogenital tract. *Seminars in diagnostic pathology*, *188*.

Ricardo-Gonzalez, R. R., Nguyen, M., Gokden, N., Sangoi, A. R., Presti Jr, J. C. & Mckenney, J. K. (2012). Plasmacytoid carcinoma of the bladder: a urothelial carcinoma variant with a predilection for intraperitoneal spread. *The Journal of urology*, *187*, 852-855.

Ro, J. Y., Shen, S. S., Lee, H. I., Hong, E. K., Lee, Y. H., Cho, N. H., Jung, S. J., Choi, Y. J. & Ayala, A. G. (2008). Plasmacytoid transitional cell carcinoma of urinary bladder: a clinicopathologic study of 9 cases. *The American journal of surgical pathology*, *32*, 752-757.

Sahin, A. A., Myhre, M., Ro, J. Y., Sneige, N., Dekmezian, R. H. & Ayala, A. G. (1991). Plasmacytoid transitional cell carcinoma. Report of a case with initial presentation mimicking multiple myeloma. *Acta Cytol*, May-Jun. *35*, 277-280.

Samaratunga, H. & Khoo, K. (2004). Micropapillary variant of urothelial carcinoma of the urinary bladder; a clinicopathological and immunohistochemical study. *Histopathology*, *45*, 55-64.

Sari, A., Uyaroglu, M. A., Ermete, M., Oder, M., Girgin, C. & Dincer, C. (2007). Microcystic urothelial carcinoma of the urinary bladder metastatic to the penis. *Pathology & Oncology Research*, *13*, 170-173.

Sato, K., Ueda, Y., Kawamura, K., Aihara, K. & Katsuda, S. (2009). Plasmacytoid urothelial carcinoma of the urinary bladder: a case report and immunohistochemical study. *Pathology, research and practice*, *205*, 189-194.

Scosyrev, E., Ely, B. W., Messing, E. M., Speights, V., Grossman, H. B., Wood, D. P., De Vere White, R. W., Vogelzang, N. J., Trump, D. L. & Natale, R. B. (2011). Do mixed histological features affect survival benefit from neoadjuvant platinum-based combination chemotherapy in patients with locally advanced bladder cancer? A secondary analysis of Southwest Oncology Group-Directed Intergroup Study (S8710). *BJU international*, *108*, 693-699.

Scosyrev, E., Yao, J. & Messing, E. (2009). Urothelial carcinoma versus squamous cell carcinoma of bladder: is survival different with stage adjustment? *Urology*, Apr. *73*, 822-827.

Shanks, J. H. & Iczkowski, K. A. (2009). Divergent differentiation in urothelial carcinoma and other bladder cancer subtypes with selected mimics. *Histopathology*, *54*, 885-900.

Shapur, N. K., Katz, R., Pode, D., Shapiro, A., Yutkin, V., Pizov, G., Appelbaum, L., Zorn, K. C., Duvdevani, M., Landau, E. H. & Gofrit, O. N. (2011). Is radical cystectomy mandatory in every patient with variant histology of bladder cancer. *Rare tumors*, Apr 4. *3*, e22.

Shokeir, A. (2004). Squamous cell carcinoma of the bladder: pathology, diagnosis and treatment. *BJU international*, *93*, 216-220.

Sim, S. J., Ro, J. Y., Ordonez, N. G., Park, Y. W., Kee, K. H. & Ayala, A. G. (1999). Metastatic renal cell carcinoma to the bladder: a clinicopathologic and immunohistochemical study. *Modern pathology: an official journal of the United States and Canadian Academy of Pathology, Inc*, 12, 351-355.

Soylu, A., Aydin, N. E., Yilmaz, U., Kutlu, R. & Gunes, A. (2005). Urothelial carcinoma featuring lipid cell and plasmacytoid morphology with poor prognostic outcome. *Urology*, Apr. *65*, 797.

Sung, M.-T., Zhang, S., Maclennan, G. T., Lopez-Beltran, A., Montironi, R., Wang, M., Tan, P.-H. & Cheng, L. (2008). Histogenesis of clear cell adenocarcinoma in the urinary tract, evidence of urothelial origin. *Clinical Cancer Research*, 14, 1947-1955.

Sung, M. T., Wang, M., Maclennan, G., Eble, J., Tan, P. H., Lopez-Beltran, A., Montironi, R., Harris, J., Kuhar, M. & Cheng, L. (2007). Histogenesis of sarcomatoid urothelial carcinoma of the urinary bladder: evidence for a common clonal origin with divergent differentiation. *The Journal of pathology*, *211*, 420-430.

Talbert, M. L. & Young, R. H. (1989a). Carcinomas of the urinary bladder with deceptively benign-appearing foci. A report of three cases. *Am J Surg Pathol*, May. *13*, 374-381.

Talbert, M. L. & Young, R. H. (1989b). Carcinomas of the urinary bladder with deceptively benign-appearing foci: a report of three cases. *The American journal of surgical pathology*, *13*, 374-381.

Tamas, E. F., Nielsen, M. E., Schoenberg, M. P. & Epstein, J. I. (2007). Lymphoepithelioma-like carcinoma of the urinary tract: a clinicopathological study of 30 pure and mixed cases. *Modern pathology*, *20*, 828-834.

Tavora, F. & Epstein, J. I. (2008). Bladder cancer, pathological classification and staging. *BJU international*, *102*, 1216-1220.

Torenbeek, R., Blomjous, C., De Bruin, P., Newling, D. & Meijer, C. (1994). Sarcomatoid carcinoma of the urinary bladder: clinicopathologic analysis of 18 cases with immunohistochemical and electron microscopic findings. *The American journal of surgical pathology*, *18*, 241-249.

Vang, R. & Abrams, J. (2000). A micropapillary variant of transitional cell carcinoma arising in the ureter. *Archives of pathology & laboratory medicine*, *124*, 1347-1348.

Volmar, K. E., Chan, T. Y., De Marzo, A. M. & Epstein, J. I. (2003). Florid von Brunn nests mimicking urothelial carcinoma: a morphologic and immunohistochemical comparison to the nested variant of urothelial carcinoma. *The American journal of surgical pathology*, *27*, 1243-1252.

Wang, J. & Wang, F. W. (2013). The Natural History, Treatment Pattern, and Outcomes of Patients With Micropapillary Bladder Carcinoma. *American journal of clinical oncology*.

Wang, J., Wang, F. W., Lagrange, C. A., Hemstreet Iii, G. P. & Kessinger, A. (2010). Clinical features of sarcomatoid carcinoma (carcinosarcoma) of the urinary bladder: analysis of 221 cases. *Sarcoma*, 2010.

Wang, J. K., Boorjian, S. A., Cheville, J. C., Kim, S. P., Tarrell, R. F., Thapa, P. & Frank, I. (2012). Outcomes following radical cystectomy for micropapillary bladder cancer versus pure urothelial carcinoma: a matched cohort analysis. *World journal of urology*, *30*, 801-806.

Wasco, M. J., Daignault, S., Bradley, D. & Shah, R. B. (2010). Nested variant of urothelial carcinoma: a clinicopathologic and immunohistochemical study of 30 pure and mixed cases. *Human pathology*, *41*, 163-171.

Wasco, M. J., Daignault, S., Zhang, Y., Kunju, L. P., Kinnaman, M., Braun, T., Lee, C. T. & Shah, R. B. (2007). Urothelial carcinoma with divergent histologic differentiation (mixed histologic features) predicts the presence of locally advanced bladder cancer when detected at transurethral resection. *Urology*, *70*, 69-74.

Westfall, D. E., Folpe, A. L., Paner, G. P., Oliva, E., Goldstein, L., Alsabeh, R., Gown, A. M. & Amin, M. B. (2009). Utility of a comprehensive immunohistochemical panel in the differential diagnosis of spindle cell lesions of the urinary bladder. *The American journal of surgical pathology*, *33*, 99-105.

Wick, M. & Swanson, P. (1993). Carcinosarcomas, current perspectives and an historical review of nosological concepts. *Seminars in diagnostic pathology*, 118-127.

Williamson, S. R., Zhang, S., Lopez-Beltran, A., Shah, R. B., Montironi, R., Tan, P.-H., Wang, M., Baldridge, L. A., Maclennan, G. T. & Cheng, L. (2011). Lymphoepithelioma-like carcinoma of the urinary bladder: clinicopathologic, immunohistochemical, and molecular features. *The American journal of surgical pathology*, *35*, 474-483.

Wright, J. L., Black, P. C., Brown, G. A., Porter, M. P., Kamat, A. M., Dinney, C. P. & Lin, D. W. (2007). Differences in survival among patients with sarcomatoid carcinoma: carcinosarcoma and urothelial carcinoma of the bladder. *The Journal of urology*, *178*, 2302-2307.

Young, R. & Zukerberg, L. (1991). Microcystic transitional cell carcinomas of the urinary bladder. A report of four cases. American *journal of clinical pathology*, *96*, 635.

Young, R. H. & Eble, J. N. (1991). Unusual forms of carcinoma of the urinary bladder. *Human pathology*, *22*, 948-965.

Young, R. H. & Oliva, E. (1996). Transitional cell carcinomas of the urinary bladder that may be underdiagnosed, a report of four invasive cases exemplifying the homology between neoplastic and non-neoplastic transitional cell lesions. *The American journal of surgical pathology*, *20*, 1448-1454.

Zhai, Q. J., Black, J., Ayala, A. G. & Ro, J. Y. (2007). Histologic variants of infiltrating urothelial carcinoma. *Arch Pathol Lab Med*, Aug. *131*, 1244-1256.

Zhang, W., Jiang, Y. X., Liu, Y., Yu, W. J., Zhao, H. & Li, Y. J. (2013). [Plasmacytoid urothelial carcinoma of the urinary bladder: a clinicopathologic study of 16 cases]. *Zhonghua bing li xue za zhi Chinese journal of pathology*, Jul. *42*, 433-437.

Zhang, X. M., Elhosseiny, A. & Melamed, M. R. (2002). Plasmacytoid urothelial carcinoma of the bladder. A case report and the first description of urinary cytology. *Acta Cytol*, Mar-Apr. *46*, 412-416.

Zukerberg, L. R., Harris, N. L. & Young, R. H. (1991). Carcinomas of the urinary bladder simulating malignant lymphoma, a report of five cases. *The American journal of surgical pathology*, *15*, 569-576.

In: Bladder Cancer
Editor: Samantha Haggerty
ISBN: 978-1-63321-666-2

Chapter 7

NOVEL THERAPEUTIC MODALITIES IN PATIENTS WITH ADVANCED OR METASTATIC UROTHELIAL CARCINOMA

Kazumasa Matsumoto*, Masaomi Ikeda, Takahiro Hirayama, Tetsuo Fujita and Masatsugu Iwamura

Department of Urology, Kitasato University School of Medicine, Japan

ABSTRACT

Cisplatin-based systemic chemotherapy is the gold standard approach for patients with advanced or metastatic urothelial carcinoma (UC). Combined chemotherapy with methotrexate, vinblastine, doxorubicin and cisplatin (MVAC), which was developed about 25 years ago, is an effective and frequently used modality for these life-threatening diseases. Recently, combined chemotherapy with gemcitabine and cisplatin (GC) has become another standard treatment for advanced UC. However, several limitations remain with MVAC and GC treatment. Long-term follow-up has revealed that overall survival or progression-free survival is poor, particularly with metastatic UC. There is no standard second-line

* For reprints and all correspondence: Kazumasa Matsumoto, M.D. Department of Urology, Kitasato University School of Medicine, 1-15-1 Kitasato, Minami-ku, Sagamihara, Kanagawa 252-0331; Phone: +81-42-778-9091; Fax: +81-42-778-9374; E-mail address: kazumasa@cd5.so-net.ne.jp.

treatment in patients with UC after the failure of cisplatin-based chemotherapy.

Multimodal treatment has become a standard of care for other kinds of malignancy. Combined chemotherapy with radiation for the treatment of advanced bladder cancer remains questionable, including whether this would eradicate local disease, eliminate potential micrometastases, and maintain the best quality of life possible without compromising survival.

In addition, new chemotherapy regimen, gemcitabine and paclitaxel, that is reacted with another antitumor mechanism will be effective for patients with advanced or metastatic UC who have previously been treated with MVAC. A gemcitabine and paclitaxel pharmacokinetic study showed that paclitaxel increased the accumulation of gemcitabine triphosphate, the active metabolite of gemcitabine

Furthermore, new approaches shall be taken, and one of them could be specific immunotherapy. A personalized peptide vaccination (PPV) protocol where at maximum four peptides were chosen from many candidate peptides based on pre-existing humoral immunity followed by vaccination. We reviewed here three novel approaches in patients with advanced or metastatic UC.

Keywords: Chemotherapy, radiation, peptide vaccination, urothelial carcinoma

INTRODUCTION

Patients with locally advanced urothelial carcinoma (UC) at diagnosis will subsequently develop regional progression or distant metastases. For these patients, chemotherapy is the treatment of choice. Cisplatin-based systemic chemotherapy is the standard approach for patients with inoperably advanced or metastatic urothelial carcinoma (UC). Combined chemotherapy of methotrexate, vinblastine, doxorubicin, and cisplatin (MVAC), which was developed about 25 years ago, is an effective and conventionally used modality for these life-threatening diseases (Sternberg et al., 1988; Sternberg et al., 1989; Loehrer et al., 1992). The good performance of MVAC was demonstrated in the initial randomized trial. Advanced UC patients were randomized to receive MVAC regimen or cisplatin alone, and the overall survival of the groups was 12.5 months and 8.2 months, respectively (Loehrer et al., 1992). In another trial, MVAC was shown to be superior to a combination treatment that consisted of cisplatin, cyclophoshamide, and doxorubicin with a high response rate and long survival; median survival was

48 weeks and 40 weeks, respectively (Logothetis et al., 1990). However, most UC patients will subsequently develop regional progression or distant metastases. The prognosis of patients with advanced or metastatic UC remains poor, with a median survival of approximately 12 months (Sternberg et al., 1989). The MVAC regimen has shown considerable toxicities, including myelosuppression and renal toxicity. There are no established therapeutic modalities, only palliative ones, for patients with progression or recurrence after MVAC is administered.

Recently, combined chemotherapy with gemcitabine and cisplatin (GC) has become another standard treatment for advanced UC. However, several limitations remain with MVAC and GC treatment. Long-term follow-up has revealed that overall survival or progression-free survival is poor, particularly with metastatic UC (Sternberg et al., 1989). There is no standard second-line treatment in patients with UC after the failure of cisplatin-based chemotherapy. Another modality for advanced or metastatic bladder cancer is external beam radiation therapy (EBRT). EBRT is a bladder-sparing treatment that has been performed for about 30 years. The local recurrence rate after EBRT alone was up to 70%, with 5-year overall survival rates from 20% to 40% (De Neve et al., 1995; Pollack et al., 1996). Interestingly, preclinical studies with bladder cancer animal models have demonstrated synergistic cytotoxicity when cisplatin was combined with concurrent EBRT (Mothersill et al., 1990). To overcome biologically aggressive advanced or metastatic UC, several investigators have recently explored the use of combined chemotherapy with radiation in an attempt to improve the results of EBRT alone. Therefore, new approaches shall be taken, and one of them could be specific immunotherapy. A personalized peptide vaccination (PPV) protocol where at maximum four peptides are chosen from many candidate peptides based on pre-existing humoral immunity followed by vaccination (Rosenberg, 1999; Novellino et al., 2005; Sharma et al., 2007; Sharma et al., 2008). We reviewed here three novel approaches in patients with advanced or metastatic UC.

Chemotherapy with External Beam Radiation Therapy

Multimodal treatment has become a standard of care for other kinds of malignancy. Combined chemotherapy with radiation for the treatment of advanced bladder cancer remains questionable, including whether this would eradicate local disease, eliminate potential micrometastases, and maintain the best quality of life possible without compromising survival. In clinical trials including cisplatin-based chemotherapy and radiation for bladder cancer, complete response (CR) was approximately 70% and 3- to 5-year overall survival was 35–83% (Shipley et al., 1987; Tester et al., 1993; Chauvet et al., 1996; Coppin et al., 1996; Kaufman et al., 2000; Rodel et al., 2002; Hagan et al., 2003; Kaufman et al., 2009). In addition, overall survival was similar to that of radical surgery in bladder cancer patients. However, these previous clinical trials mainly consisted of patients with organ-confined diseases. We examined the tolerability of combined MVAC with radiation and to access the efficacy in patient with locally advanced or metastatic bladder cancer.

The radiotherapy combined with MVAC treatment produces an 80% response rate with a manageable toxicity profile for locally advanced or metastatic UC patients (Ikeda et al., 2011). CR was confirmed in 13 patients (43%) and 11 patients (37%) showed partial response. The median overall survival and progression-free survival were 25.5 months and 12.8 months, respectively. The median survival time of 13 patients with CR was 37.1 months (range, 6.9–38.0 months). According to multivariate Cox proportional hazards regression analysis, good PS, CR, and four cycles of MVAC were significant predictors of progression-free survival (P = 0.025, 0.001, and 0.005, respectively). One limitation of this study is that efficacy and tolerability data for this chemoradiotherapy were evaluated retrospectively and not in a randomized trial. Our sample size was small for analysis, and we could not distribute a quality-of-life questionnaire for chemoradiotherapy. Although there was no significant predictor in terms of overall survival according to multivariate analysis, 13 patients (43%) who were treated with this chemoradiotherapy showed CR and 24 patients (80%) had major responses. In addition, they had significantly prolonged survival compared to non-responding patients. This regimen may be effective and safe for patients with advanced or metastatic bladder cancer.

In the Radiation Therapy Oncology Group (RTOG) 89-03 study (Shipley et al., 1998), 123 patients with T2–T4a bladder cancer were randomly assigned to receive either two cycles of chemotherapy followed by 64.8 Gy of EBRT with concomitant use of cisplatin or only chemo-radiation without prior chemotherapy. There were no significant differences in regard to 5-year overall survival, rates of distant metastasis, and survival with a functioning bladder in both arms. However, combining chemotherapy with radiotherapy was based on several rationales. Autopsy data show that micrometastases are often present in patients with invasive bladder cancer. One study examined autopsies from 367 pateints with muscle-invasive bladder cancer (pT2–pT4) and identified distant metastases in 68%; the frequency of metastases increased with tumor stage (pT2, 36%; pT3a, 45%; pT3b, 69%; pT4, 79%) (Wallmeroth et al., 1999). The rationale of induction chemotherapy is to treat initially present micrometastasis (Lin et al., 2009). In addition, systemic chemotherapy is tolerated better before the irradiation of cancer lesions than after local therapy (Shipley et al., 1998; Hagan et al., 2003). Furthermore, chemotherapy coupled with radiation may add the therapeutic effect of reducing the rate of distant failures. Second, drug resistance to cytotoxic agents may be related to spontaneous mutations in cancer cells, which occurs more often in tumors of greater mass (Goldie et al., 1979). Third, hypoxic cells exist in solid tumors with poor vascularity and are likely to be resistant to the treatment, especially to radiation. However, these cells may be more sensitive to the combined effects of cytotoxic agents and radiotherapy (Kennedy, 1987). Reoxygenation in hypoxic tumor cells, which increases the radiosensitivity, may occur after induction chemotherapy and result in tumor shrinkage. Fourth, radiotherapy can induce vascular sclerosis, which causes reduced access of chemotherapy agents to tumor sites (Basavaraju et al., 2002). The administration of chemotherapy before post-radiation sclerosis could increase chemoresponsiveness. Finally, certain chemotherapy drugs, such as 5-fluorouracil, cisplatin, gemcitabine, and paclitaxel, have been reported to react as radiosensitizers, which render malignant tissues more sensitive to radiation (Bentzen et al., 2007).

Several studies have reported on the prognostic factors in patients with invasive bladder cancer who were treated with chemoradiotherapy. Coppin et al. reported that low clinical staging (T2–T3a versus T3b–T4) was the independent prognostic factor of overall survival and progression-free survival (Coppin et al., 1996). Rodel et al. showed that low clinical stage and complete transurethral resection had the strongest impact on overall survival (Rodel et al., 2002). In addition, Arias et al. demonstrated that the significant factors for overall survival were T2 stage and absence of hydronephrosis (Arias et al., 2000). Thus, several studies showed that low clinical stage was a significant factor for survival.

The clinical applicability of this chemoradiotherapy is supported by the outpatient administration and a tolerable toxicity profile in previously treated patients. In the RTOG 89-03 study (Shipley et al., 1998), grade 3 or higher febrile neutropenia during the two cycles of methotrexate, cisplatin, and vinblastine was observed in 23% of patients, and lethal complication from neutropenia and sepsis occurred in three patients. Arias et al. reported that the severe adverse events following MVAC included alopecia (30%), leucopenia (16%), vomiting (12%), and thrombocytopenia (4%), while concomitant chemoradiotherapy showed severe cystitis (12%), diarrhea (4%), and leucopenia (4%) (Arias et al., 2000). Although, in our study, patients with grade 3–4 neutropenia were frequently seen, these patients were safely treated with granulocyte-colony stimulating factor and none of them had severe infections (Ikeda et al., 2011). In addition, no severe hematologic toxicities were found in patients treated with a half dose of MVAC chemotherapy with radiation. With regard to nonhematological toxicities, only one patient experienced hemorrhagic radiation cystitis 1 year after radiotherapy.

2ND LINE CHEMOTHERAPY

Gemcitabine, an analog of cytarabine, is a pyrimidine antimetabolite. The antitumor effect of gemcitabine is mediated by the inhibition of DNA synthesis. Single-agent gemcitabine has demonstrated a response rate of 23%–28% (Stadler et al., 1997; Sternberg, 2000).(Stadler et al., 1997; Sternberg, 2000)(Stadler et al., 1997; Sternberg, 2000) Paclitaxel is an anti-mitotic spindle drug that promotes microtubular aggregation and interferes with such cellular functions as mitosis cell transport and cell motility. Single-agent paclitaxel was shown to have an overall response rate of 42% in previously untreated UC (Roth et al., 1994). To separate the mechanism of antitumor efficacy, gemcitabine and paclitaxel may have complementary cytotoxicity when administered as combination therapy. In previous reports, this combination therapy showed an overall response rate of 38% to 69% and a complete response rate of 7% to 50% in previously treated and chemo-naive patient; it maintains an excellent toxicity profile (Meluch et al., 2001; Sternberg et al., 2001; Kaufman et al., 2004; Li et al., 2005; Fechner et al., 2006).

Many previous trials that assessed gemcitabine and paclitaxel (GP) regimen have demonstrated a variable response rate of 30% to 69% (Meluch et al., 2001; Sternberg et al., 2001; Kaufman et al., 2004; Li et al., 2005; Fechner et al., 2006; Takahashi et al., 2006; Suyama et al., 2009). However, treatment strategies varied for the first-line or the second-line setting. For the second-line treatment, Suyama et al. reported that the overall response rate was 33% and the disease control rate was 73%, with median overall survival of 11.3 months (Suyama et al., 2009). Sternberg et al. reported that overall response rate of an every 2-week regimen was 60%, and median overall survival was 14.4 months (Sternberg et al., 2001). Recently in a randomized phase III trial, Albers et al. reported on the results of an every 3 weeks GP chemotherapy (short-term arm) versus an every 3 weeks GP chemotherapy until disease progression (prolonged arm) (Albers et al., 2011). Overall survival was lower in both arms, with a median survival of 7.8 months for the short-term arm and 8.0 months for the prolonged arm. However, the overall response rate was 37.5% and 41.5%, respectively. These reports demonstrated therapeutic effects consistent with our results. How this regimen compares with other described regimens, including a variety of dose and treatment courses for patients with MVAC refractory cancer, is difficult to evaluate given the limited number of patients in this trial. Combined GP chemotherapy may possibly be useful for patients who were previously treated with cisplatin-based chemotherapy. We demonstrated that the GP regimen produces a 37% overall response rate and a 71% disease control rate with a tolerable toxicity profile as a second-line chemotherapy for advanced or metastatic UC patients who have previously been treated with MVAC chemotherapy (Ikeda et al., 2011). The median overall survival and progression-free survival were 12.4 and 6.1 months, respectively. In addition, 1-year survival was 52% after MVAC treatment failed. The limitation of this study is that data about better safety and tolerability of gemcitabine and paclitaxel were not collected with the quality of life (QOL) questionnaires. QOL questionnaires were not disease or treatment specific, and they did not address specific toxicities for chemotherapy such as mucositis and neutropenic sepsis, which are of particular concern in the treatment of cancer. However, 9 patients who were treated with the MVAC regimen showed high tolerability for gemcitabine and paclitaxel chemotherapy. Another limitation is that omitting the dose on days 8 and 15 may have decreased myelosuppression, as it may have enabled more courses to start on schedule and allowed patients to have a break from treatment every third week.

A gemcitabine and paclitaxel pharmacokinetic study reported that paclitaxel increased the accumulation of gemcitabine triphoshate, the active metabolite of gemcitabine (Shord et al., 2003). Previous trials that assessed this combination regimen have demonstrated a variable response rate of 38% to 69% (Meluch et al., 2001; Sternberg et al., 2001; Kaufman et al., 2004; Li et al., 2005; Fechner et al., 2006). Fechner et al examined chemotherapy as a second-line treatment for advanced bladder cancer (Fechner et al., 2006). However, how this regimen compares to other described regimen, including a variety of dose and treatment courses for patients with MVAC refractory cancer, is difficult to evaluate given the limited number of patients in this trial. On the other hand, Kaufmann et al reported that the treatment effect of gemcitabine and paclitaxel as a first-line therapy was less than expected with more standard MVAC or gemcitabine and cisplatin (Kaufman et al., 2004). The combination of gemcitabine and paclitaxel would be useful only for patients who were previously treated with cisplatin-based chemotherapy.

The clinical applicability of GP regimen is supported by the outpatient administration and a tolerable toxicity profile in previously treated patients. Meluch et al. reported that the severe adverse events following GP treatment included leukopenia (46%), anemia (28%) and thrombocytopenia (13%) (Meluch et al., 2001). Febrile neutropenia occurred in 10 patients (19%), and one patient (2%) had treatment-related death. In our study no life-threatening complications were seen (Ikeda et al., 2011). While grade 3–4 neutropenia was frequently seen, these patients were safely treated using G-CSF and none had severe infections. Severe pulmonary toxicities such as interstitial pneumonitis were reported in another study (Li et al., 2005). However, none of the 24 patients experienced pulmonary toxicities, even though one patient received 12 cycles of GP treatment. Although it is not clear if pulmonary toxicities occur in a dose-dependent manner, these complications are more likely to occur with high-dose regimens (Dunsford et al., 1999).

Multidrug resistance (MDR) of tumors is frequently associated with decreased cellular accumulation of anticancer drugs. Therefore, it is of importance to investigate the correlation between MDR gene expression and cisplatin resistance (Choi et al., 2006). Hoffmann et al. reported that high *MDR1* and excision repair cross-complementing 1 (*ERCC1*) gene expression was associated with inferior outcome after cisplatin-based chemotherapy for locally advanced bladder cancer (Hoffmann et al., 2010). According to this mechanism, a MVAC non-responder would show resistance to the GP chemotherapy. As new drugs such as gemcitabine and paclitaxel have been introduced to the management of UC, biomarkers including MDR1 and ERCC1 would be required to select appropriate treatment options for individualized patient care.

Peptide Vaccination

A personalized peptide vaccination (PPV) protocol where at maximum four peptides are chosen from many candidate peptides based on pre-existing humoral immunity followed by vaccination (Rosenberg, 1999; Novellino et al., 2005; Sharma et al., 2007; Sharma et al., 2008). The recently conducted randomized clinical trial of PPV for advanced prostate cancer patients showed the favorite clinical responses in the vaccinated group (Noguchi et al., 2010), whereas the vast majority of the randomized cancer vaccine trials failed to obtain better clinical responses in vaccine group (Finke et al., 2007; Goldman et al., 2009). We addressed the feasibility of PPV to advanced UC patients who failed to MVAC therapy in phase I study by employing a new protocol, a twelve consecutive weekly administration of PPV without any additional chemotherapy because expected survival time of those patients (Matsumoto et al., 2011).

No major adverse events were observed in any of ten patients entered, although all the patients developed grade 1 or 2 local dermatological reactions at the injection sites. Therefore, in terms of safety, the toxicity of the twelve-consecutive weekly PPV regimen was tolerable and acceptable for MVAC-refractory UC patients.

With regard to peptide-induced immune reactions, an increase in peptide-specific IFN-γ production in response to at least one of the four vaccinated peptides was observed in the majority of post-vaccination PBMC (8 of 9 cases), regardless of no (n=5) or lower (n=5) levels of CTL activity in pre-vaccination PBMC. It is of note that the boosted CTL activities to all the four peptides were seen in the post-vaccination samples of CR case. Similarly, an increase of peptide-specific IgG was observed in the post-vaccination plasma of the majority of patients (8 of 9 cases). There were more than 10 (n=7) and 100-fold increases (n=6) of IgG levels in the post-vaccination samples, suggesting that clonal expansion of peptide-reactive B cells was induced by this regimen.

These results indicated that both the cellular and humoral responses were well boosted in the vast majority of UC patients under this regimen. The profile of positive peptides varied greatly from a patient to a patient, suggesting that peptides suitable for use in each patient are different, in consistent with the previously reported results in the other types of cancers (Rosenberg, 1999; Novellino et al., 2005; Sharma et al., 2007; Sharma et al., 2008). This would be in part due to both heterogeneity of tumor nature and immunological diversity of tumor-reactive CTL in each patient.

Although cellular immunity is the predominant effecter arm of antitumor responses, humoral immunity also plays an important role in host defense against cancer cells (Valmori et al., 2007). One possible explanation is that pre-existing CD4 Th1 cells specific to the vaccinated peptides facilitate peptide-specific antibody production as well as CTL induction. Alternatively, some peptides may bind both class I and class II HLA and induce activation of CTL and Th1 cells (Harada et al., 2004). Biological roles of peptide-reactive IgG are also needed to be clarified in near future.

The overall response rate defined as radiological imaging is comparable to those seen in previous reported studies of combined chemotherapy such as gemcitabine and paclitaxel (Uhm et al., 2007; Han et al., 2008). The median survival time of the 10 patients was somewhat lower than that reported with those chemotherapy regimens (Uhm et al., 2007; Han et al., 2008), the responders to peptide vaccination showed a median survival time of 24 months. One possible reason for the prolonged survival in the present study may be the UC extremely sensitive for immunotherapy.

Massive infiltration of CD45RO+ cells into tumor sites of a PR patient after PPV, whereas they were resided around vessels and connective tissues before vaccination. PPV induced infiltration of CD45RO+ lymphocytes, but neither CD8+ T cells nor CD20+ B cells, in tumor sites of prostate cancer patients (Noguchi et al., 2007). In contrast, a large numbers of CD45RA+ cells were found in lymphoid follicles near tumor sites after PPV, while they were scarcely observed around vessels before vaccination. In considering that CD45RO expression in activated or memory T cells and CD45RA expression in naïve T cells (Clement, 1992), PPV induced infiltration of CD45RO+ activated/memory CD4+ T cells into tumor sites and also accumulation of CD45RA naïve CD4+ T cells in lymphoid follicles near tumor sites.

Conclusion

Vinflunine is a new microtubule inhibitor that has activity against UC. Bellmunt reported that a randomized phase III study of vinflunine and best supportive care (BSC) versus BSC alone in the treatment of patients with advanced UC who had experienced progression after a first-line platinum-containing regimen (Bellmunt et al., 2009). The median overall survival was significantly longer for vinflunine and BSC than BSC alone (6.9 and 4.3 months, respectively) ($p=0.04$). Although administration of vinflunine for survival benefit was significant, prolongation of valuable life time was approximately 2 months. Exclusively having one published data, it is very difficult for us to lead to the conclusion that vinflunine is a formal second-line chemotherapeutic regimen.

Gemicitabine and cisplatin (GC) treatment became first-line chemotherapy instead of MVAC treatment. In GC era, following chemotherapeutic regimen, including the second-line chemotherapy, is more difficult. Further improvement of new modalities for advanced or metastatic UC would likely also have the advantages of either increasing efficacy or decreasing toxicity, which would lead to higher QOL and would be determined chemotherapeutic dose and treatment days. The response observed with new therapeutic modalities which were shown in this review will require the confirmation of larger numbers of patients who have been previously treated with cisplatin-based chemotherapy. Further investigation is warranted, but this review suggests an immediate role for new therapeutic options in this patient group.

REFERENCES

Albers P, Park SI, Niegisch G, et al (2011). Randomized phase III trial of 2nd line gemcitabine and paclitaxel chemotherapy in patients with advanced bladder cancer: short-term versus prolonged treatment [German Association of Urological Oncology (AUO) trial AB 20/99]. *Ann. Oncol.*, 22, 288-94.

Arias F, Dominguez MA, Martinez E, et al (2000). Chemoradiotherapy for muscle invading bladder carcinoma. Final report of a single institutional organ-sparing program. *Int. J. Radiat. Oncol. Biol. Phys.*, 47, 373-8.

Basavaraju SR, Easterly CE (2002). Pathophysiological effects of radiation on atherosclerosis development and progression, and the incidence of cardiovascular complications. *Med. Phys.*, 29, 2391-403.

Bellmunt J, Theodore C, Demkov T, et al (2009). Phase III trial of vinflunine plus best supportive care compared with best supportive care alone after a platinum-containing regimen in patients with advanced transitional cell carcinoma of the urothelial tract. *J. Clin. Oncol.*, 27, 4454-61.

Bentzen SM, Harari PM, Bernier J (2007). Exploitable mechanisms for combining drugs with radiation: concepts, achievements and future directions. *Nat. Clin. Pract. Oncol.*, 4, 172-80.

Chauvet B, Brewer Y, Felix-Faure C, et al (1996). Concurrent cisplatin and radiotherapy for patients with muscle invasive bladder cancer who are not candidates for radical cystectomy. *J. Urol.*, 156, 1258-62.

Choi MK, Kim DD (2006). Platinum transporters and drug resistance. *Arch. Pharm. Res.*, 29, 1067-73.

Clement LT (1992). Isoforms of the CD45 common leukocyte antigen family: markers for human T-cell differentiation. *J. Clin. Immunol.*, 12, 1-10.

Coppin CM, Gospodarowicz MK, James K, et al (1996). Improved local control of invasive bladder cancer by concurrent cisplatin and preoperative or definitive radiation. The National Cancer Institute of Canada Clinical Trials Group. *J. Clin. Oncol.*, 14, 2901-7.

De Neve W, Lybeert ML, Goor C, et al (1995). Radiotherapy for T2 and T3 carcinoma of the bladder: the influence of overall treatment time. *Radiother Oncol*, 36, 183-8.

Dunsford ML, Mead GM, Bateman AC, et al (1999). Severe pulmonary toxicity in patients treated with a combination of docetaxel and gemcitabine for metastatic transitional cell carcinoma. *Ann. Oncol.*, 10, 943-7.

Fechner G, Siener R, Reimann M, et al (2006). Randomised phase II trial of gemcitabine and paclitaxel second-line chemotherapy in patients with transitional cell carcinoma (AUO Trial AB 20/99). *Int. J. Clin. Pract.*, 60, 27-31.

Finke LH, Wentworth K, Blumenstein B, et al (2007). Lessons from randomized phase III studies with active cancer immunotherapies--outcomes from the 2006 meeting of the Cancer Vaccine Consortium (CVC). *Vaccine*, 25 Suppl 2, B97-B109.

Goldie JH, Coldman AJ (1979). A mathematic model for relating the drug sensitivity of tumors to their spontaneous mutation rate. *Cancer Treat Rep*, 63, 1727-33.

Goldman B, DeFrancesco L (2009). The cancer vaccine roller coaster. *Nat. Biotechnol.*, 27, 129-39.

Hagan MP, Winter KA, Kaufman DS, et al (2003). RTOG 97-06: initial report of a phase I-II trial of selective bladder conservation using TURBT, twice-daily accelerated irradiation sensitized with cisplatin, and adjuvant MCV combination chemotherapy. *Int. J. Radiat. Oncol. Biol. Phys.*, 57, 665-72.

Han KS, Joung JY, Kim TS, et al (2008). Methotrexate, vinblastine, doxorubicin and cisplatin combination regimen as salvage chemotherapy for patients with advanced or metastatic transitional cell carcinoma after failure of gemcitabine and cisplatin chemotherapy. *Br. J. Cancer*, 98, 86-90.

Harada M, Gohara R, Matsueda S, et al (2004). In vivo evidence that peptide vaccination can induce HLA-DR-restricted CD4+ T cells reactive to a class I tumor peptide. *J. Immunol.*, 172, 2659-67.

Hoffmann AC, Wild P, Leicht C, et al (2010). MDR1 and ERCC1 expression predict outcome of patients with locally advanced bladder cancer receiving adjuvant chemotherapy. *Neoplasia*, 12, 628-36.

Ikeda M, Matsumoto K, Niibe Y, et al (2011). The radiotherapy with methotrexate, vinblastine, doxorubicin, and cisplatin treatment is an effective therapeutic option in patients with advanced or metastatic bladder cancer. *J. Radiat. Res.*, 52, 674-9.

Ikeda M, Matsumoto K, Tabata K, et al (2011). Combination of gemcitabine and paclitaxel is a favorable option for patients with advanced or metastatic urothelial carcinoma previously treated with cisplatin-based chemotherapy. *Jpn J. Clin. Oncol.*, 41, 1214-20.

Kaufman DS, Carducci MA, Kuzel TM, et al (2004). A multi-institutional phase II trial of gemcitabine plus paclitaxel in patients with locally advanced or metastatic urothelial cancer. *Urol. Oncol.*, 22, 393-7.

Kaufman DS, Winter KA, Shipley WU, et al (2000). The initial results in muscle-invading bladder cancer of RTOG 95-06: phase I/II trial of transurethral surgery plus radiation therapy with concurrent cisplatin and 5-fluorouracil followed by selective bladder preservation or cystectomy depending on the initial response. *Oncologist*, 5, 471-6.

Kaufman DS, Winter KA, Shipley WU, et al (2009). Phase I-II RTOG study (99-06) of patients with muscle-invasive bladder cancer undergoing transurethral surgery, paclitaxel, cisplatin, and twice-daily radiotherapy followed by selective bladder preservation or radical cystectomy and adjuvant chemotherapy. *Urology*, 73, 833-7.

Kennedy KA (1987). Hypoxic cells as specific drug targets for chemotherapy. *Anticancer Drug Des*, 2, 181-94.

Li J, Juliar B, Yiannoutsos C, et al (2005). Weekly paclitaxel and gemcitabine in advanced transitional-cell carcinoma of the urothelium: a phase II Hoosier Oncology Group study. *J. Clin. Oncol.*, 23, 1185-91.

Lin CC, Hsu CH, Cheng JC, et al (2009). Induction cisplatin and fluorouracil-based chemotherapy followed by concurrent chemoradiation for muscle-invasive bladder cancer. *Int. J. Radiat. Oncol. Biol. Phys.*, 75, 442-8.

Loehrer PJ, Sr., Einhorn LH, Elson PJ, et al (1992). A randomized comparison of cisplatin alone or in combination with methotrexate, vinblastine, and doxorubicin in patients with metastatic urothelial carcinoma: a cooperative group study. *J. Clin. Oncol.*, 10, 1066-73.

Logothetis CJ, Dexeus FH, Finn L, et al (1990). A prospective randomized trial comparing MVAC and CISCA chemotherapy for patients with metastatic urothelial tumors. *J. Clin. Oncol.*, 8, 1050-5.

Matsumoto K, Noguchi M, Satoh T, et al (2011). A phase I study of personalized peptide vaccination for advanced urothelial carcinoma patients who failed treatment with methotrexate, vinblastine, adriamycin and cisplatin. *BJU Int.*, 108, 831-8.

Meluch AA, Greco FA, Burris HA, 3rd, et al (2001). Paclitaxel and gemcitabine chemotherapy for advanced transitional-cell carcinoma of the urothelial tract: a phase II trial of the Minnie pearl cancer research network. *J. Clin. Oncol.*, 19, 3018-24.

Mothersill C, Seymour CB, Cusack A, et al (1990). The effect of radiation and cytotoxic platinum compounds on the growth of normal and tumour bladder explant cultures. *Acta Oncol.*, 29, 179-84.

Noguchi M, Mine T, Komatsu N, et al (2010). Assessment of immunological biomarkers in patients with advanced cancer treated by personalized peptide vaccination. *Cancer Biol. Ther.*, 10, 1266-79.

Noguchi M, Yao A, Harada M, et al (2007). Immunological evaluation of neoadjuvant peptide vaccination before radical prostatectomy for patients with localized prostate cancer. *Prostate*, 67, 933-42.

Novellino L, Castelli C, Parmiani G (2005). A listing of human tumor antigens recognized by T cells: March 2004 update. *Cancer Immunol. Immunother*, 54, 187-207.

Pollack A, Zagars GZ (1996). Radiotherapy for stage T3b transitional cell carcinoma of the bladder. *Semin. Urol. Oncol.*, 14, 86-95.

Rodel C, Grabenbauer GG, Kuhn R, et al (2002). Combined-modality treatment and selective organ preservation in invasive bladder cancer: long-term results. *J. Clin. Oncol.*, 20, 3061-71.

Rosenberg SA (1999). A new era for cancer immunotherapy based on the genes that encode cancer antigens. *Immunity*, 10, 281-7.

Roth BJ, Dreicer R, Einhorn LH, et al (1994). Significant activity of paclitaxel in advanced transitional-cell carcinoma of the urothelium: a phase II trial of the Eastern Cooperative Oncology Group. *J. Clin. Oncol.*, 12, 2264-70.

Sharma P, Bajorin DF, Jungbluth AA, et al (2008). Immune responses detected in urothelial carcinoma patients after vaccination with NY-ESO-1 protein plus BCG and GM-CSF. *J. Immunother*, 31, 849-57.

Sharma P, Shen Y, Wen S, et al (2007). CD8 tumor-infiltrating lymphocytes are predictive of survival in muscle-invasive urothelial carcinoma. *Proc. Natl. Acad. Sci. USA*, 104, 3967-72.

Shipley WU, Prout GR, Jr., Einstein AB, et al (1987). Treatment of invasive bladder cancer by cisplatin and radiation in patients unsuited for surgery. *JAMA*, 258, 931-5.

Shipley WU, Winter KA, Kaufman DS, et al (1998). Phase III trial of neoadjuvant chemotherapy in patients with invasive bladder cancer treated with selective bladder preservation by combined radiation therapy and chemotherapy: initial results of Radiation Therapy Oncology Group 89-03. *J. Clin. Oncol.*, 16, 3576-83.

Shord SS, Faucette SR, Gillenwater HH, et al (2003). Gemcitabine pharmacokinetics and interaction with paclitaxel in patients with advanced non-small-cell lung cancer. *Cancer Chemother Pharmacol.*, 51, 328-36.

Stadler WM, Kuzel T, Roth B, et al (1997). Phase II study of single-agent gemcitabine in previously untreated patients with metastatic urothelial cancer. *J. Clin. Oncol.*, 15, 3394-8.

Sternberg CN (2000). Gemcitabine in bladder cancer. *Semin. Oncol.*, 27, 31-9.

Sternberg CN, Calabro F, Pizzocaro G, et al (2001). Chemotherapy with an every-2-week regimen of gemcitabine and paclitaxel in patients with transitional cell carcinoma who have received prior cisplatin-based therapy. *Cancer*, 92, 2993-8.

Sternberg CN, Yagoda A, Scher HI, et al (1989). Methotrexate, vinblastine, doxorubicin, and cisplatin for advanced transitional cell carcinoma of the urothelium. Efficacy and patterns of response and relapse. *Cancer*, 64, 2448-58.

Sternberg CN, Yagoda A, Scher HI, et al (1988). M-VAC (methotrexate, vinblastine, doxorubicin and cisplatin) for advanced transitional cell carcinoma of the urothelium. *J. Urol.*, 139, 461-9.

Suyama T, Ueda T, Fukasawa S, et al (2009). Combination of gemcitabine and paclitaxel as second-line chemotherapy for advanced urothelial carcinoma. *Jpn J. Clin. Oncol.*, 39, 244-50.

Takahashi T, Higashi S, Nishiyama H, et al (2006). Biweekly paclitaxel and gemcitabine for patients with advanced urothelial cancer ineligible for cisplatin-based regimen. *Jpn J. Clin. Oncol.*, 36, 104-8.

Tester W, Porter A, Asbell S, et al (1993). Combined modality program with possible organ preservation for invasive bladder carcinoma: results of RTOG protocol 85-12. *Int. J. Radiat. Oncol. Biol. Phys.*, 25, 783-90.

Uhm JE, Lim HY, Kim WS, et al (2007). Paclitaxel with cisplatin as salvage treatment for patients with previously treated advanced transitional cell carcinoma of the urothelial tract. *Neoplasia*, 9, 18-22.

Valmori D, Souleimanian NE, Tosello V, et al (2007). Vaccination with NY-ESO-1 protein and CpG in Montanide induces integrated antibody/Th1 responses and CD8 T cells through cross-priming. *Proc. Natl. Acad. Sci. USA*, 104, 8947-52.

Wallmeroth A, Wagner U, Moch H, et al (1999). Patterns of metastasis in muscle-invasive bladder cancer (pT2-4): An autopsy study on 367 patients. *Urol. Int.*, 62, 69-75.

INDEX

I

J

K

L

M

N

O

P

Q

R

S

T

U

V

W

X

Y

Z